Regenerative Engineering
Advanced Materials Science Principles

CRC PRESS SERIES IN
REGENERATIVE ENGINEERING

SERIES EDITOR
Cato T. Laurencin
University of Connecticut Health Center, Farmington, Connecticut

PUBLISHED TITLES

Regenerative Engineering: Advanced Materials Science Principles
Yusuf Khan and Cato T. Laurencin

3D Bioprinting in Regenerative Engineering:
Principles and Applications
Ali Khademhosseini and Gulden Camci-Unal

Regenerative Engineering and Developmental Biology:
Principles and Applications
David M. Gardiner

Regenerative Engineering
Advanced Materials Science Principles

Edited by
Yusuf Khan and Cato T. Laurencin

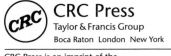

CRC Press is an imprint of the
Taylor & Francis Group, an **informa** business

CRC Press
Taylor & Francis Group
6000 Broken Sound Parkway NW, Suite 300
Boca Raton, FL 33487-2742

First issued in paperback 2023

© 2018 by Taylor & Francis Group, LLC
CRC Press is an imprint of Taylor & Francis Group, an Informa business

No claim to original U.S. Government works

ISBN 13: 978-1-03-265232-0 (pbk)
ISBN 13: 978-1-4987-3824-8 (hbk)
ISBN 13: 978-1-315-12107-9 (ebk)

DOI: 10.1201/9781315121079

Publisher's Note
The publisher has gone to great lengths to ensure the quality of this reprint but points out that some imperfections in the original copies may be apparent.

**Visit the Taylor & Francis Web site at
www.taylorandfrancis.com**

**and the CRC Press Web site at
www.crcpress.com**

Contents

Contributors

Mary Badon
Department of Orthopaedic Surgery
University of Connecticut Health Center
Farmington, Connecticut

Arijit Bhattacharjee
Department of Biological Sciences and
    Bioengineering
Indian Institute of Technology Kanpur
Kanpur, Uttar Pradesh, India

Karen J. L. Burg
College of Veterinary Medicine
University of Georgia
Athens, Georgia

Nathan J. Castro
Department of Mechanical and Aerospace
    Engineering
The George Washington University
Washington, District of Columbia

Junqiu Cheng
National Engineering Research Center for
    Biomaterials
Sichuan University
Chengdu, China

Haitao Cui
Department of Mechanical and Aerospace
    Engineering
The George Washington University
Washington, District of Columbia

Meng Deng
Department of Agricultural and Biological
    Engineering
Purdue University
West Lafayette, Indiana

Steven E. Ellis
Division of Biological Infrastructure,
    Biological Sciences Directorate
National Science Foundation
Arlington, Virginia

Hongsong Fan
National Engineering Research Center for
    Biomaterials
Sichuan University
Chengdu, China

Cheryl T. Gomillion
College of Engineering
University of Georgia
Athens, Georgia

Dhirendra S. Katti
Department of Biological Sciences and
    Bioengineering
Indian Institute of Technology Kanpur
Kanpur, Uttar Pradesh, India

Yusuf Khan
Department of Orthopaedic Surgery
University of Connecticut Health Center
Farmington, Connecticut

Liangju Kuang
Department of Agricultural and Biological
Engineering
Purdue University
West Lafayette, Indiana

Cato T. Laurencin
Department of Orthopaedic Surgery
University of Connecticut Health Center
Farmington, Connecticut
and
Raymond and Beverly Sackler Center for
Biomedical, Biological, Physical and
Engineering Sciences
Farmington, Connecticut
and
Department of Materials Science &
Engineering
University of Connecticut
Storrs, Connecticut

Se-Jun Lee
Department of Mechanical and Aerospace
Engineering
The George Washington University
Washington, District of Columbia

Paul A. Lengemann
Department of Agricultural and Biological
Engineering
Purdue University
West Lafayette, Indiana

Xiangfeng Li
National Engineering Research Center for
Biomaterials
Sichuan University
Chengdu, China

Mengqian Liu
Department of Bioengineering
University of California
San Diego, California

Garima Lohiya
Department of Biological Sciences and
Bioengineering
Indian Institute of Technology Kanpur
Kanpur, Uttar Pradesh, India

Aman Mahajan
Department of Biological Sciences and
Bioengineering
Indian Institute of Technology Kanpur
Kanpur, Uttar Pradesh, India

Naveen Nagiah
Institute for Regenerative Engineering
University of Connecticut Health Center
Farmington, Connecticut

M. Sriram
Department of Biological Sciences and
Bioengineering
Indian Institute of Technology Kanpur
Kanpur, Uttar Pradesh, India

Shyni Varghese
Department of Bioengineering
University of California
San Diego, California

Lijie G. Zhang
Departments of Mechanical and Aerospace
Engineering, Biomedical Engineering,
and Medicine
The George Washington University
Washington, District of Columbia

Xingdong Zhang
National Engineering Research Center for
Biomaterials
Sichuan University
Chengdu, China

Changchun Zhou
National Engineering Research Center for
    Biomaterials
Sichuan University
Chengdu, China

Wei Zhu
Department of Mechanical and Aerospace
    Engineering
The George Washington University
Washington, District of Columbia

CHAPTER 1

Regenerative Engineering

Advanced Materials Science Principles

Mary Badon and Yusuf Khan

University of Connecticut Health Center

CONTENTS

1.1 INTRODUCTION

Regenerative engineering is a field of study that focuses on the development of novel materials and the redevelopment of existing materials to facilitate the growth and the development of tissues and complete structures. It differentiates itself from regenerative medicine, which primarily focuses on the biologic process and the growth/development of a single type of tissue, rather than on complex tissues and structures.[1]

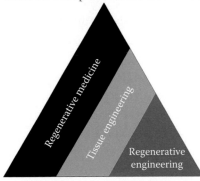

A variety of materials have been recently developed and refined, including polymers, ceramics, metals, as well as nano, micro, and macro scale composites and scaffolds. The goal is to create materials that guide the development of tissues through transient physical and biochemical development cues with minimal long-term effects on the biologic system due to either delayed or unpredictable degradation of the material itself or a transition into biologic senescence and inertness. This book aims to provide a comprehensive overview of the advances in the field related specifically to the development and utilization of materials, define their role in the biomedical sciences, and provide context for their innovations.[2–5]

1.2 TISSUE REGENERATION AND THE ROLE OF REGENERATIVE ENGINEERING

Regeneration mimics the natural processes of tissue formation. Tissues normally form during embryonic tissue formation, tissue growth and development (fetal and postnatal), remodeling (degradation-formation), and healing (repair vs. regeneration). Regenerative engineering focuses on using cues from the earlier tissue formation periods and applies them to those that occur later in hopes of directing adult tissue away from simple repair, where a defect in the tissue fills with relatively biologically inactive, nonfunctional scar, and toward regeneration, where the defect or injury fills with tissue that is indistinguishable from the original tissue.[6]

Tissue gaps or large scars present biological challenges. For example, infarcts secondary to pulmonary emboli or myocardial infarctions result in relatively noncompliant scars taking the place of biologically active tissues that not only reduce the overall function of the organ because the scar cannot carry out the role of the organ but also impede the function of the rest of the organ due to physical forces restricting the dynamic movement of the tissue. These gaps or scars can be focused in a single area, as in the case of infarction, but they can also be diffusely distributed in the native, normal tissue, as in the case of infection. Classically, in the case of hand cellulitis, the compliance of the soft tissues is reduced after the infection has cleared, resulting in joint capsule stiffness as well as generation restriction throughout the skin and muscle, thereby resulting in restricted range of motion and discomfort.

Regenerative engineering seeks to create physical solutions for biological defects. Ideally, implants are engineered so that they create the appropriate and optimally timed biological and physical signals to the surrounding tissues to stimulate the formation of bioidentical tissues that are continuous with the surrounding biological environment. The implants simultaneously act as templates and guides for tissue growth.[7] The choice of materials and the nature in which they are assembled can have dramatic impacts on this process. Several chapters within this volume discuss this impact through the relationship between cells and materials of different content, structure, and scale.

When a regenerative engineering problem is approached, the engineers must decide what strategy they would like to employ for regeneration. Namely, would they like to recapitulate developmental conditions with appropriate cells and/or extracellular matrices or if the engineers would instead provide conditions (cells and matrix) that favor tissue formation from the surrounding adult tissue? One approach would be to establish the growth of tissues, most often within scaffolds, in a petri dish or *in vitro*. This approach is an important testing ground to establish the feasibility and the presence of appropriate developmental biochemical cues, such as growth factors that can be controlled, but it is an approach with limitations and does not fully recapitulate the *in vivo* environment. Other challenges present themselves, however, when trying to approach tissue regeneration problems *in vivo*.

The emphasis within regenerative engineering is to take advantage of the biological environment and mechanical stimuli in the *in vivo* settings in combination with implants that utilize the advances in materials engineering, signal transduction, and surgical techniques to facilitate the growth of complex tissues and structures to both increase the scope of medical problems that can be addressed and minimize the duration of time that tissue regeneration takes by simultaneously growing multiple types of tissue, rather than needing sequential reconstructive procedures. Through the formation of implants using advanced biomaterials and techniques, the regenerative engineer is setting the stage for tissue growth and development to occur *in vivo*, rather than solely in a petri dish.

1.3 THE CLINICAL RELEVANCE AND IMPORTANCE OF REGENERATIVE ENGINEERING

The evolution of regenerative engineering can be marked by examples of similar efforts over time. The field can trace its origins through related efforts in the 1970s and 1980s when ntegra™ (Integra Lifesciences Corporation, Plainsboro, New Jersey, USA), a collagen-glycosaminoglycan (GAG) matrix that is used to help complex wounds and burns heal, first emerged. Manufactured in the form of a wound dressing that is placed over a debrided wound, the collagen-GAG scaffold provides the needed structure for angiogenesis and ingrowth of dermal skin cells to remodel the damaged site. During the course of 14–21 days, as fibroblasts and mesenchymal stem cells migrate into the scaffold, the collagen scaffold is resorbed and replaced with the patient's own tissue and the wound is gradually healed. This breakthrough resulted in a user-friendly product that was rapidly integrated into clinical practice and is routinely used today.[8–10]

Several tissue engineering technologies that have been developed over that time span have been applied to medicine. For example, scaffolds have been used for skin and bone regeneration.[11,12] However, these tissues have the innate ability to regenerate and the injuries in which scaffolds have been used. In these cases, the scaffolds were used to overcome the limitations on normal healing that were introduced by the physical size of the injury rather than to stimulate the development of new tissues that do not possess some regeneration capacity on their own. Examples of tissues that spontaneously regenerate include bone, epithelia (including stomach lining, intestinal lining, and skin), and smooth muscle. The areas of active research in tissues that do not spontaneously regenerate include articular cartilage, ligaments (predominantly collagen type I), intervertebral discs of the spine, cardiac muscle, skeletal muscle, and nerves[13–15] and also those tissues that do regenerate like bone but can fail to heal due to injury severity or related pathology.

Bone is a highly structured and dynamic tissue, which consists of organic and inorganic matrices and is both innervated and vascularized as it regenerates. However, factors such as the size of defects (defects or gaps >2 mm are at risk of not healing), unfavorable environments such as the collapse of tissues into defects precluding healing in the case of periodontal defects, and inappropriate physical forces across the injured area in the case of unstable or over-stabilized fractures resulting in hypertrophic or atrophic nonunions (an ideal strain is thought to be 2% for bone healing to occur).[16]

Collagen type I is predominantly found in ligaments. The *in vivo* regeneration of ligaments like the anterior cruciate ligament (ACL) presents a considerable challenge as the intra-articular environment in which the ACL also accommodates articular cartilage, which has very different regeneration requirements. The synovial fluid provides the articular cartilage with the necessary nutrition and lubrication and also presents an obstacle to ligament healing. Polymers such as poly(lactic acid), especially when combined with biologics like bone morphogenetic protein and other growth factors, provide soft tissue reconstruction solutions for both articular cartilage and ligaments in the intra-articular milieu.[17–19]

Current trends in the United States suggest that regenerative engineering advances in ACL reconstruction are timely. Between 1994 and 2006, the population-adjusted estimate of the rate of ACL reconstructions increased by 37% (33.0/100,000 capita or 86,837 total procedures to 45.1/100,000 capita or 134,421 total procedures).[20] Synthetic ACL grafts would provide a reasonable option for patients who (1) prefer to not undergo tissue harvest and avoid the associated donor site morbidity associated with hamstring or patellar tendon harvest, (2) wish to avoid the small, but real risk of disease transmission and higher graft failure rates associated with donor grafts (allograft), and (3) require revision surgery due to previous ACL graft reconstruction failures in the setting of autografts or allografts.

1.4 THE ROLE OF ADVANCED MATERIALS SCIENCE PRINCIPLES IN REGENERATIVE ENGINEERING

This volume covers the latest advances in the use of metals and ceramics for regenerative engineering. As opposed to soft tissue reconstruction, where goals can be set for the graft to be fully integrated into the surrounding native tissue, ceramics and metals have been used to replace tissues. The evolution of biomaterials in this context can be divided into generations: first generation (bioinert materials), second generation (bioactive and biodegradable materials), and third generation (materials designed to stimulate specific responses at the molecular level).[21]

Metals and ceramics are particularly interesting materials in that they have been used as implant materials for generations, but they are still the topic of considerable research, and new advancements are made every day. In the 1950s and 1960s, metals and ceramics were used because they provided surfaces that were relatively biologically inert and permanent. Materials like stainless steel were used by Charnley in the late 1950s in the form of a cemented total hip arthroplasty to create the first joint replacements.[22] At that time, the view was that materials had to be durable because of the significant forces across joints and because of the long-term survival factor regarding the implant in the human body, which harbors a highly corrosive environment. Corrosion of the implant would present two problems. Degradation of the metal/ceramic implant would change the implant's physical characteristics and surface texture, and could also release ions or other chemicals into the bloodstream and affect distant parts of the body.

The individual components of stainless steel constitute a good material for joint replacement implants. The chromium, while corrosive on its own, when paired with oxygen in the form of Cr_2O_3, creates a highly corrosion resistant oxide coating. The most common type of stainless steel used for implants is austenitic steel, which contains stabilizing elements like nickel or manganese.[21]

While stainless steel is still commonly used in the trauma setting, joint replacement implants have evolved to use other metallic alloys like titanium and cobalt chromium. The cobalt chromium alloy can also be made austenitic. These alloys have superior mechanical properties, for instance a yield stress more similar to the native tissue, to facilitate bone health and prevent its loss due to stress shielding. This is an example of how a scientific advance in materials can contribute to the biology of bone.[21]

First-generation ceramics include alumina, zirconia, as well as porous ceramics whose physical structure facilitated bone ingrowth. Alumina, in the form of α-AL_2O_3, was first reported in 1972 as a component of a femoral head in joint arthroplasty.[20] Ceramic materials were later used for acetabular cups.[23-26] They demonstrated low wear rates, resistance to corrosion, high strength, and good biocompatibility compared to previous acetabular cups made of polyethylene. Despite these favorable characteristics and improved biocompatibility compared to polyethylene, which shed particles that would result in osteolysis, ceramic acetabular cups had low fracture toughness resulting in catastrophic failures. Currently, ceramics like alumina and zirconia are used for total joint arthroplasty in conjunction with other types of materials such as ceramic femoral heads with polyethylene liners.[21,27,28]

Porous ceramics intuitively would provide an opportunity for native tissues to integrate into the structure of the scaffold. For example, the calcium carbonate structure of certain corals mimics trabecular bone. Additionally, alumina and zirconia can be made into porous forms with foaming agents that produce gases while the ceramic is setting. These experiments, however, led to disappointing results given the risk of mechanical collapse, predicted by the Ryshkewitch equation, ($\sigma = \sigma_0 \cdot e^{-cp}$).[29]

However, the advent of three-dimensional printing created new possibilities for the use of ceramics with superstructures. One of the problems with porous ceramics is that they were too brittle and would fail catastrophically under stress. This does not happen in normal bone because the combination of inorganic hydroxyapatite (approximately 65%) and organic components like collagen (approximately 10%) would add elasticity and flexibility.[29]

Additionally, the three-dimensional printer allows reproduction of the hierarchical patterns that help bone withstand factoring by dissipating energy, minimizing localized damage rather than using a foaming agent that creates a random but relatively uniform pattern of pores. The current utility of 3-D printing is constantly growing, and is discussed in this volume.

Hierarchal patterns are common in nature. Bone has two characteristic patterns: dense cortical bone as well as trabecular bone (also referred to as cancellous or spongy bone). The relatively heavy cortical bone provides strength and is load bearing. Cortical bone has a porosity of approximately 3.5%. Its thickness and density vary according to the amount of force that is imparted on it, referred to as Wolff's law with higher load bearing bones like the femur having thicker and denser cortical bone than the upper extremities. In addition to being responsive to mechanical forces, the cortical bone has a complex microstructure, including canals and conduits for blood supply, innervation, and cell-to-cell communication between osteocytes, and providing specialized pores for cells involved in bone turnover like osteoblasts and osteoclasts.[30]

The trabecular bone with its honeycomb-like structure is contained within the cortical bone shell. A trabecula (plural trabeculae, from Latin for "small beam") is a small, often microscopic, tissue element in the form of a small beam, strut, or rod. The rod and beam structure of the trabecular bone, in contrast to the denser cortical bone, creates a lightweight network of cavities within the bone. The trabecular bone is less dense with approximately 79.3% porosity. This reflects its function in the body. The trabecular bone does contribute to the overall strength of the bone and it also provides space for both fatty and red bone marrow as well as blood cell production.[4,30]

Beginning in the 1970s, scientists began to explore the use of natural coral graft substitutes that are derived from the exoskeleton of marine madreporic corals as bone xenograph.[31] The structural unit of coral, referred to as porites, is similar to that of cancellous bone both in their scaffold-like network of channels and cavities as well as some of their mechanical properties. Consisting of primarily calcium carbonate, coral proved to be biocompatible, relatively inert, osteoconductive by providing channels for blood vessel ingrowth, and bioresorbable. Coral can be treated using a hydrothermal process to convert it to a non-resorbable hydroxyapatite material.[15] The primary advantage of using corals as a source of bone graft over laboratory-made ceramics and composites is their similarity in hierarchical structure to cadaver bone. Coralline grafts are neither osteoinductive nor osteogenic unless combined with other biologics like bone morphogenetic protein (BMP). They are primarily sold as calcified matrix.[24,31]

Other sources of natural xenograft, surprisingly, are trees. In 2009, Italian scientists announced a breakthrough in the use of wood as a bone substitute. Like bone, trees and other vascularized plants contain a hierarchal microstructure consisting of channels that bring water and sap up and down the organism through canals called xylem and phloem. A hydroxyapatite scaffold is made from native wood using a sequence of thermal and hydrothermal chemical processes in five steps, including pyrolysis of ligneous raw materials, carburization to yield calcium carbide, oxidation to transform calcium carbide to calcium oxide, carbonation by hydrothermal process under CO_2 pressure to yield calcium carbonate (the same component in untreated coralline xenografts), and finally, phosphatization using hydrothermal treatment to achieve hydroxyapatite. Despite the caustic nature of some of these reactions, they yield an innovative inorganic biomorphic scaffold providing a biomimetic nanostructure surface for orthopedic and engineering applications. The inventors of this wood-derived, hydroxyapatite scaffold claimed that their material will permit better penetration during bone growth and allow more flexion than metal or hard ceramic grafts.[32] This example demonstrates that scientists can look to nature for inspiration and ways to repurpose materials that evolved to serve other purposes.[32]

Three-dimensional printing can overcome the limitations of using natural tissues. Markus Buehler of the Department of Civil and Environmental Engineering at the Massachusetts Institute of Technology generated "metamaterials" to create new advancements in manufacturing materials, tissue engineering, electrical circuits, and more. This group combined design, computational modeling, and 3-D assembly with chemistry, materials engineering, and tissue engineering to generate entirely new "metamaterials" that are then printed into novel structures using a 3-D printer. In other words, materials can be combined, and new structures can be designed to generate scaffolds that today do not exist in either engineered or biological forms. These metamaterials can be chemically or physically resurfaced to interact and direct the growth of surrounding tissues, even degrade at predetermined rates, have complex structures including channels and pores to direct the development of structures like blood vessels and nerves, and have specific physical and mechanical behaviors.[33]

The freedom offered by computer design, microengineering, and 3-D printing may be necessary for the formation of scaffolds to be capable of inducing complex tissue regeneration. This would include the growth of gradient tissues and structures like joints which consist of multiple types of tissue, and cell- and growth factor-based tissue engineering where signaling molecules can be geographically localized to materials, yielding "intelligent" scaffolds that can direct the growth and behavior of the surrounding native tissue. This can include stimulating ingrowth of the surrounding native tissue and directing the development of local stem cells in the local native tissue to yield new tissue types distinct from the surrounding tissues.[7,34]

Scaffolds can also be made to direct the behavior of surrounding cells by modifying their surface characteristics and their ultrastructure in the case of nanofibers, or by including growth factors and biologics. Growth factors that have been surface adsorbed or encapsulated in scaffolds include VGEF, PDGF, EGF, and BMP. These scaffolds can then trigger angiogenesis, bone formation, and fibroblast ingrowth. The method of cross-linking or embedding growth factors onto or into scaffolds can control the timing of their release into the surrounding tissues.[11,15,34–36]

Physical factors, such as the ultrastructure of a scaffold, can influence cell behavior just as dramatically as signal transduction and growth factors. The advances in textiles and materials science have given rise to electrospinning as a fiber production method (discussed in detail in this volume), which uses electric force to draw charged threads of polymer solutions or polymer melts up to fiber diameters in the order of some hundred nanometers. Working with polymers of this scale creates a very large surface area to volume ratio (this ratio for a nanofiber can be as large as 103 times that of a microfiber), increases flexibility in surface functionalities and superior mechanical performance (e.g., stiffness and tensile strength) compared with other materials and scaffolds made with the same type of polymer.[37–39]

These fibers can then be further woven into scaffolds with precise and complicated structures that can influence cell behavior. These nanofiber scaffolds can be so finely engineered that they have morphological similarities to the native extracellular matrix. Nanoscale alterations in scaffold topography elicit diverse cell behavior, ranging from changes in cell adhesion, motility, activation of specific signal transduction cascades, such as tyrosine kinases, and can even lead to the upregulation or downregulation of gene expression. For example, skeletal muscle can be cultured *in vitro*; however, if the fibers are not oriented systematically, the resulting tissue will not be functional. A nanoscale polycaprolactone scaffold can be constructed and seeded with myoblasts, which then orient themselves in a uniform pattern as well as change their morphology with a larger length to diameter ratio, which is compatible with force production characteristic of skeletal muscle tissue.[40]

1.5 SUMMARY

Methods from the fields of materials science, computer design, textiles, cell biology, and translational medicine are all applied to common conditions that occur in the human because of aging, trauma, or disease in regenerative engineering. Current frontiers focus on not only tissue propagation but more sophisticated questions which involve function, development, and a focus on structure regeneration as opposed to individual tissues. A well-designed material, scaffold, or implant has immediate applications in the clinical world as physicians and surgeons seek to improve patient outcomes as well as patient experiences to minimize the duration and number of interventions necessary to restore structure and function. This volume, *Regenerative Engineering: Advanced Materials Science Principles*, seeks to discuss a number of materials, methods, applications, and interactions that are of interest to the regenerative engineer. As the field continues to grow, so will the potential applications of advanced materials and materials science and the myriad novel ways they can be applied to complex tissue repair.

REFERENCES

1. Martino, S.; D'Angelo, F.; Armentano, I.; Kenny, J. M.; Orlacchio, A. Stem cell-biomaterial interactions for regenerative medicine. *Biotechnol. Adv.* **2012**, *30* (1), 338–351. DOI: 10.1016/j.biotechadv.2011.06.015.
2. Yu, X.; Tang, X.; Gohil, S. V.; Laurencin, C. T. Biomaterials for bone regenerative engineering. *Adv. Healthcare Mater.* **2015**, *4* (9), 1268–1285. DOI: 10.1002/adhm.201400760.
3. Hamadouche, M.; Sedel, L. Ceramics in orthopaedics. *J. Bone Joint Surg. Br.* **2000**, *82* (8), 1095–1099.
4. Khan, Y. M.; Katti, D. S.; Laurencin, C. T. Novel polymer-synthesized ceramic composite-based system for bone repair: an in vitro evaluation. *J. Biomed. Mater. Res. A* **2004**, *69* (4), 728–737. DOI: 10.1002/jbm.a.30051.
5. Ambrosio, A. M.; Sahota, J. S.; Khan, Y.; Laurencin, C. T. A novel amorphous calcium phosphate polymer ceramic for bone repair: I. Synthesis and characterization. *J. Biomed. Mater. Res.* **2001**, *58* (3), 295–301.
6. Qazi, T. H.; Mooney, D. J.; Pumberger, M.; Geißler, S.; Duda, G. N. Biomaterials based strategies for skeletal muscle tissue engineering: existing technologies and future trends. *Biomaterials* **2015**, *53*, 502–521. DOI: 10.1016/j.biomaterials.2015.02.110.
7. Jiang, T.; Carbone, E. J.; Lo, K. W.-H.; Laurencin, C. T. Electrospinning of polymer nanofibers for tissue regeneration. *Prog. Polym. Sci.* **2015**, *46*, 1–24. DOI: 10.1016/j.progpolymsci.2014.12.001.
8. Place, E. S.; Evans, N. D.; Stevens, M. M. Complexity in biomaterials for tissue engineering. *Nat. Mater.* **2009**, *8* (6), 457–470. DOI: 10.1038/nmat2441.
9. Barnes, C. P.; Sell, S. A.; Boland, E. D.; Simpson, D. G.; Bowlin, G. L. Nanofiber technology: designing the next generation of tissue engineering scaffolds. *Adv. Drug Deliv. Rev.* **2007**, *59* (14), 1413–1433. DOI: 10.1016/j.addr.2007.04.022.
10. Pérez, R. A.; Won, J.-E.; Knowles, J. C.; Kim, H.-W. Naturally and synthetic smart composite biomaterials for tissue regeneration. *Adv. Drug Deliv. Rev.* **2013**, *65* (4), 471–496. DOI: 10.1016/j.addr.2012.03.009.

11. Lu, W.; Ji, K.; Kirkham, J.; Yan, Y.; Boccaccini, A. R.; Kellett, M.; Jin, Y.; Yang, X. B. Bone tissue engineering by using a combination of polymer/bioglass composites with human adipose-derived stem cells. *Cell Tissue Res.* **2014**, *356* (1), 97–107. DOI: 10.1007/s00441-013-1770-z.

12. Cushnie, E. K.; Khan, Y. M.; Laurencin, C. T. Amorphous hydroxyapatite-sintered polymeric scaffolds for bone tissue regeneration: physical characterization studies. *J. Biomed. Mater. Res. A* **2008**, *84* (1), 54–62. DOI: 10.1002/jbm.a.31380.

13. Zhang, Z.; Rouabhia, M.; Wang, Z.; Roberge, C.; Shi, G.; Roche, P.; Li, J.; Dao, L. H. Electrically conductive biodegradable polymer composite for nerve regeneration: electricity-stimulated neurite outgrowth and axon regeneration. *Artif. Organs* **2007**, *31* (1), 13–22. DOI: 10.1111/j.1525-1594.2007.00335.x.

14. Hyatt, J.-P. K.; Roy, R. R.; Baldwin, K. M.; Wernig, A.; Edgerton, V. R. Activity-unrelated neural control of myogenic factors in a slow muscle. *Muscle Nerve* **2006**, *33* (1), 49–60. DOI: 10.1002/mus.20433.

15. Campana, V.; Milano, G.; Pagano, E.; Barba, M.; Cicione, C.; Salonna, G.; Lattanzi, W.; Logroscino, G. Bone substitutes in orthopaedic surgery: from basic science to clinical practice. *J. Mater. Sci. Mater. Med.* **2014**, *25* (10), 2445–2461. DOI: 10.1007/s10856-014-5240-2.

16. Amini, A. R.; Adams, D. J.; Laurencin, C. T.; Nukavarapu, S. P. Optimally porous and biomechanically compatible scaffolds for large-area bone regeneration. *Tissue Eng. Part A* **2012**, *18* (13–14), 1376–1388. DOI: 10.1089/ten.TEA.2011.0076.

17. Font Tellado, S.; Rosado Balmayor, E.; Van Griensven, M. Strategies to engineer tendon/ligament-to-bone interface: biomaterials, cells and growth factors. *Adv. Drug Deliv. Rev.* **2015**, 1–15. DOI: 10.1016/j.addr.2015.03.004.

18. Subramanian, A.; Krishnan, U. M.; Sethuraman, S. Axially aligned electrically conducting biodegradable nanofibers for neural regeneration. *J. Mater. Sci. Mater. Med.* **2012**, *23* (7), 1797–1809. DOI: 10.1007/s10856-012-4654-y.

19. Liang, D.; Hsiao, B. S.; Chu, B. Functional electrospun nanofibrous scaffolds for biomedical applications. *Adv. Drug Deliv. Rev.* **2007**, *59* (14), 1392–1412. DOI: 10.1016/j.addr.2007.04.021.

20. Buller, L. T.; Best, M. J.; Baraga, M. G.; Kaplan, L. D. Trends in anterior cruciate ligament reconstruction in the United States. *Orthop. J. Sport. Med.* **2015**, *3* (1), 232596711456366. DOI: 10.1177/2325967114563664.

21. Mahyudin, F.; Widhiyanto, L.; Hermawan, H. Biomaterials in orthopaedics. *Adv. Struct. Mater.* **2016**, *58* (July), 161–181. DOI: 10.1007/978-3-319-14845-8_7.

22. Charnley, J. Anchorage of the femoral head prosthesis to the shaft of the femur. *J. Bone Joint Surg. Br.* **1960**, *42–B*, 28–30.

23. Hench, L. L. The story of bioglass. *J. Mater. Sci. Mater. Med.* **2006**, *17* (11), 967–978. DOI: 10.1007/s10856-006-0432-z.

24. Xynos, I. D.; Hukkanen, M. V; Batten, J. J.; Buttery, L. D.; Hench, L. L.; Polak, J. M. Bioglass 45S5 stimulates osteoblast turnover and enhances bone formation in vitro: implications and applications for bone tissue engineering. *Calcif. Tissue Int.* **2000**, *67* (4), 321–329. DOI: 10.1007/s002230001134.

25. Hench, L. L. Bioceramics. *J. Am. Ceram. Soc.* **2005**, *81* (7), 1705–1728. DOI: 10.1111/j.1151-2916.1998.tb02540.x.

26. Roether, J.; Gough, J. E.; Boccaccini, A. R.; Hench, L. L.; Maquet, V.; Jérôme, R. Novel bioresorbable and bioactive composites based on bioactive glass and polylactide foams for bone tissue engineering. *J. Mater. Sci. Mater. Med.* **2002**, *13* (12), 1207–1214.

27. Rezwan, K.; Chen, Q. Z.; Blaker, J. J.; Boccaccini, A. R. Biodegradable and bioactive porous polymer/inorganic composite scaffolds for bone tissue engineering. *Biomaterials* **2006**, *27* (18), 3413–3431. DOI: 10.1016/j.biomaterials.2006.01.039.

28. Audebert, P. Recent trends in polypyrrole electrochemistry, nanostructuration, and applications. In: Cosnier S.; Karyakin A., editors, *Electropolymerization: Concepts, Materials and Applications*. Weinheim, Germany: Wiley-VCH Verlag GmbH & Co. KGaA, **2010**.

29. Ryshkewitch, E. Compression strength of porous sintered alumina and zirconia. *J. Am. Ceram. Soc.* **1953**, *36* (2), 65–68.

30. Renders, G. A. P.; Mulder, L.; van Ruijven, L. J.; van Eijden, T. M. G. J. Porosity of human mandibular condylar bone. *J. Anat.* **2007**, *210* (3), 239–248. DOI: 10.1111/j.1469–7580.2007.00693.x.

31. Demers, C.; Hamdy, C. R.; Corsi, K.; Chellat, F.; Tabrizian, M.; Yahia, L. Natural coral exoskeleton as a bone graft substitute: a review. *Biomed. Mater. Eng.* **2002**, *12* (1), 15–35.

32. Tampieri, A.; Sprio, S.; Ruffini, A.; Celotti, G.; Lesci, I. G.; Roveri, N. From wood to bone: multi-step process to convert wood hierarchical structures into biomimetic hydroxyapatite scaffolds for bone tissue engineering. *J. Mater. Chem.* **2009**, *19* (28), 4973. DOI: 10.1039/b900333a.

33. Qin, Z.; Jung, G. S.; Kang, M. J.; Buehler, M. J. The mechanics and design of a lightweight three-dimensional graphene assembly. *Sci. Adv.* **2017**, *3* (1), e1601536. DOI: 10.1126/sciadv.1601536.

34. Jabbarzadeh, E.; Deng, M.; Lv, Q.; Jiang, T.; Khan, Y. M.; Nair, L. S.; Laurencin, C. T. VEGF-incorporated biomimetic poly(lactide-co-glycolide) sintered microsphere scaffolds for bone tissue engineering. *J. Biomed. Mater. Res. B. Appl. Biomater.* **2012**, *100* (8), 2187–2196. DOI: 10.1002/jbm.b.32787.

35. Matthews, B. G.; Torreggiani, E.; Roeder, E.; Matic, I.; Grcevic, D.; Kalajzic, I. Osteogenic potential of alpha smooth muscle actin expressing muscle resident progenitor cells. *Bone* **2016**, *84*, 69–77. DOI: 10.1016/j.bone.2015.12.010.

36. Jabbarzadeh, E.; Nair, L. S.; Khan, Y. M.; Deng, M.; Laurencin, C. T. Apatite nano-crystalline surface modification of poly(lactide-co-glycolide) sintered microsphere scaffolds for bone tissue engineering: implications for protein adsorption. *J. Biomater. Sci. Polym. Ed.* **2007**, *18* (9), 1141–1152. DOI: 10.1163/156856207781554073.

37. Huang, Z.-M.; Zhang, Y.-Z.; Kotaki, M.; Ramakrishna, S. A review on polymer nanofibers by electrospinning and their applications in nanocomposites. *Compos. Sci. Technol.* **2003**, *63* (15), 2223–2253. DOI: 10.1016/S0266–3538(03)00178-7.

38. Li, M.; Guo, Y.; Wei, Y.; MacDiarmid, A. G.; Lelkes, P. I. Electrospinning polyaniline-contained gelatin nanofibers for tissue engineering applications. *Biomaterials* **2006**, *27* (13), 2705–2715. DOI: 10.1016/j.biomaterials.2005.11.037.

39. Yang, F.; Murugan, R.; Wang, S.; Ramakrishna, S. Electrospinning of nano/micro scale poly(L-lactic acid) aligned fibers and their potential in neural tissue engineering. *Biomaterials* **2005**, *26* (15), 2603–2610. DOI: 10.1016/j.biomaterials.2004.06.051.

40. Tang, X.; Khan, Y.; Laurencin, C. T. Electroconductive nanofiber scaffolds for muscle regenerative engineering. *Front. Bioeng. Biotechnol.* DOI: 10.3389/conf.FBIOE.2016.01.02165.

CHAPTER 2

Polymeric Hydrogels via Click Chemistry for Regenerative Engineering

Liangju Kuang, Paul A. Lengemann, and Meng Deng

Purdue University

CONTENTS

2.1 INTRODUCTION

Regenerative engineering is a rapidly evolving interdisciplinary field with the ultimate objective of creating complex tissues and tissue interfaces based on the convergence of tissue engineering, advanced materials science, stem cell science, and developmental biology [1]. Tissue regeneration efficacy is considerably dependent on having a biomaterial scaffold that can mimic natural extracellular matrix (ECM) and promote desired cell-matrix interactions. The interactions between cells and scaffolds greatly influence cell functions, such as adhesion, proliferation, migration, and differentiation, which are the hallmarks of regenerative engineering. The capacity of cells to sense and respond to a microenvironment (niche) is critical to how they develop and function within tissues. A variety of physical, chemical, and biological cues presented by the microenvironment act as important regulators of cell fate and function [1, 2].

Hydrogels composed of polymeric networks swollen in water have been widely investigated as three-dimensional (3D) scaffolds that mimic natural ECM and provide mechanical, spatial, and biological signals for regulating and guiding a desirable cellular response. Hydrogels possess many attractive properties, such as cytocompatibility, tissue mimetic water content, support of cellular activities, sustained release of growth factors, controllable physical properties, and minimally invasive surgical delivery via injection in a liquid phase [2].

Many methods, such as noncovalent physical interaction and covalent chemical cross-linking, have already been employed for the preparation of hydrogels [2]. In 2001, Sharpless introduced click chemistry to describe reactions that are high yielding, wide in scope, stereospecific, and simple to perform and only create by-products that can be removed without chromatography and that can be conducted in easily removable or benign solvents [3]. Since then, click chemistry has provided a versatile platform for the design and fabrication of hydrogels as engineered cell niches because it allows for cell encapsulations while simultaneously providing a 3D environment mimicking the extracellular environment of natural tissues. It also allows for the effective modulation of physiochemical and biological properties of hydrogels. Such control is beneficial for the development of cell-instructive hydrogels and the regeneration of tissues characterized by cell heterogeneity and anisotropic properties. In particular, the recent developments of copper-free click chemistry, such as metal-free [3+2] cycloaddition, thiol-ene chemistry, Diels–Alder reaction, aldehyde-hydrazide click reaction, and oxime click reaction, show great promise to form hydrogels due to the lack of potentially toxic catalysts or immunogenic enzymes [4]. This chapter presents an overview of recent exciting developments in click hydrogels and their applications for regenerative engineering.

2.2 AZIDE-ALKYNE CYCLOADDITION

2.2.1 CuAAC Click Reaction

Since the first reports in 2001 by Kolb, Finn, and Sharpless the copper(I)-catalyzed alkyne-azide cycloaddition (CuAAC) click reaction has been perceived as ideal for chemical synthesis, drug discovery, bioconjugation, and biochemistry because of its fast reaction rate, high efficiency, excellent regiospecificity, and bioorthogonality [3]. The CuAAC reaction proceeds by [3+2] cycloaddition between an azide and an alkyne to form 1, 2, 3-triazole (Figure 2.1) [4]. Some macromolecules, including poly(vinyl alcohol) [5], polyethylene glycol (PEG) [6–8], cellulose [9], and hyaluronan (HA) [10, 11], have been modified with pendant acetylene and azide groups to form hydrogels by the CuAAC reaction. Table 2.1 shows an overview of representative synthetic hydrogels formed through click reactions for regenerative engineering. Generally, hydrogels prepared via CuAAC have controlled architectures

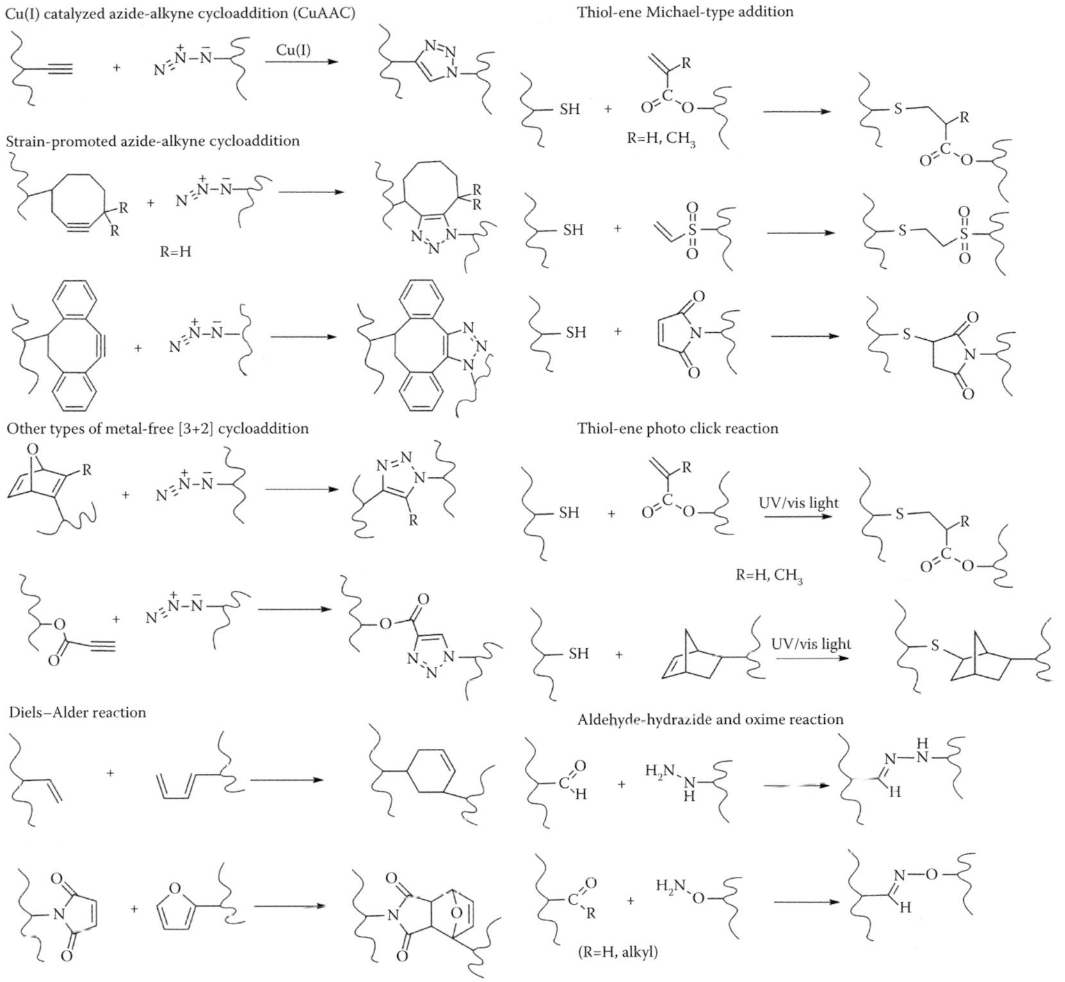

FIGURE 2.1 Overview and classification of click reactions.

TABLE 2.1 Overview of Representative Synthetic Hydrogels Formed through Click Reactions for Regenerative Engineering

Composition	Preparation Method	Application	Reference
A tetra-acetylene terminated 4-arm PEG, PEG diazide	CuAAC	Cell delivery	[6]
Hyaluronic acid (HA), gelatin, and chondroitin sulfate (CS)	CuAAC	Support the adhesion and proliferation of chondrocytes	[11]
Azide-modified HA and cyclooctyne-modified HA	SPAAC	*In vitro* cell encapsulation	[12]
Azido-modified PEG and cyclooctyne-modified PEG	SPAAC	Cell encapsulation	[13]
Oxanorbornadiene functionalized chitosan, azido functionalized HA	SPAAC	Human ASC encapsulation	[14]

(Continued)

TABLE 2.1 *(Continued)* Overview of Representative Synthetic Hydrogels Formed through Click Reactions for Regenerative Engineering

Composition	Preparation Method	Application	Reference
Azide-functionalized chitosan and propiolic acid ester-functional PEG	Copper-free click chemistry	Support hMSC attachment and proliferation	[15]
Thiolated-heparin and acrylate-ended PEG	Visible-light-initiated Thiol-ene photo click	3T3 fibroblast encapsulation and epidermal growth factor delivery	[16]
Norbornene-functionalized PEG and cysteine-containing peptides	Thiol-ene photo click	Culture embryonic stem cell-derived motor neurons	[17]
4-arm PEG norbornene, PEG-dithiol, and matrix metalloproteinase	Thiol-ene photo click	hMSC encapsulation, valvular interstitial cells	[18–20]
HA-SH and PEGDA	Michael-type addition	Network connectivity and cell adhesion	[11, 21]
RGD modified multiarm PEG and trifunctional protease sensitive cross-linking peptide	Michael-type addition	Human bone marrow stromal cell line, HS-5 cell encapsulation	[22]
PEG-4MAL, or PEG-4A, or PEG-4VS, and RGD	Michael-type addition	C2C12 cell encapsulation	[23]
Acrylated HA/4 arm PEG-SH	Michael-type addition	Bone regeneration	[24]
HA-SH and 4-arm PEG-VS	Michael-type addition	Cartilage tissue engineering	[25]
PEG-8MAL or PEG-4MAL, or PEG-4VS, and RGD	Michael-type addition	Human dermal fibroblasts cell encapsulation	[26]
PEG methacrylate and thiolated chitosan	Michael-type addition via UV lamp irradiation	L929 cell encapsulation, tissue adhesive	[27]
HA-furan and dimaleimide PEG (PEG-2MAL)	Diels–Alder	Cell encapsulation and articular cartilage tissue repair	[28]
Furan and tyramine functionalized HA and PEG-2MAL	Enzymatic crosslinking and Diels–Alder click chemistry	Cartilage tissue engineering	[29]
HA-furan and PEG-2MAL	Diels–Alder	Tissue engineering, emulate ECM	[30–32]

(Continued)

TABLE 2.1 *(Continued)* Overview of Representative Synthetic Hydrogels Formed through Click Reactions for Regenerative Engineering

Composition	Preparation Method	Application	Reference
HA-furan and HA-maleimide	Diels–Alder	Deliver dexamethasone for adipose tissue	[33]
HA-furan, HA-maleimide, and Fe_3O_4 nanospheres conjugated HA	Diels–Alder	Deliver dexamethasone for adipose tissue	[34]
HA-furan, gelatin-furan, PEG-2MAL, and CS	Diels–Alder and then EDC/NHS crosslinking	Cartilage	[35]
Glycol chitosan and multi-benzaldehyde functionalized PEG analogues	Aldehyde-hydrazide	Chondrocyte encapsulation, cartilage tissue engineering	[36]
Hydrazide-modified poly(L-glutamic acid) and Aldehyde-modified alginate	Aldehyde-hydrazide	Chondrocyte encapsulation, cartilage tissue engineering	[37]
Furan and ADH functionalized HA, furan and aldehyde functionalized HA	Diels–Alder and Aldehyde-hydrazide	Cartilage tissue engineering	[38]
HA-ADH/four-armed aminooxy-PEG (PEG-4AO) hydrogel, Alginate-ADH/PEG-4AO hydrogel, and PEG-4AO/4-arm ketone-PEG hydrogel	Oxime cross-linking	Catheter	[39]

and improved mechanical properties. *In vitro* cell culture studies showed that resulting hydrogels were capable of supporting cell adhesion and proliferation [6, 11]. Although the versatility of CuAAC has been broadly exploited for hydrogels, the toxicity of the copper catalyst and the concomitant need for additional purification have raised concerns and somewhat restricted the use of the conjugation reaction in biomaterials applications.

2.2.2 SPAAC Click Reaction

There has been a strong interest in the development of metal-free bioclick reactions. In one of its earliest reports, the Bertozzi group introduced strain-promoted alkyne-azide cyclo-addition (SPAAC), which proceeded without the need for a copper catalyst by instead using ring strain and electron withdrawing fluorine substituents [40]. Takahashi *et al.* chemically modified HA with azide (HA–N_3) and cyclooctyne groups (HA–C), respectively. Aqueous HA–N_3 and HA–C solutions cross-linked rapidly via SPAAC without any catalyst under physiological conditions. Although the hydrogel possessed good biocompatibility after intraperitoneal and subcutaneous administration, it displayed fast hydrolytic degradation, which may hamper its application in tissue engineering; in a cell culture media with fetal bovine serum, the hydrogel degraded within only 4 days [12]. Zhong *et al.* successfully prepared a PEG hydrogel via SPAAC between azido-modified PEG and cyclooctyne-modified PEG. An *in vitro* cytotoxicity assay of the hydrogel showed that the cell viability was above 85% after a 48-hour incubation period. *In vivo* studies also verified good biocompatibility of the hydrogel. The hydrogel, formed *in situ* after a subcutaneous injection in Kungming mice, caused a mild inflammatory response with the surrounding tissues fully recovering one week after injection [13]. However, the hydrogel also demonstrated pH-dependent hydrolysis and fast degradability, resulting from ester groups in the cross-linked network. Overall, SPAAC is gaining widespread attention for use in the preparation of *in situ*-forming hydrogels since the microenvironment within the hydrogel scaffold can be precisely manipulated spatially and temporally; however, it also possesses synthetic challenges in the multistep preparation of the ring-strained alkyne.

2.2.3 Other Types of Metal-Free [3+2] Cycloaddition

More recently, oxanorbornadiene (OB) moieties have been considered to be effective functional molecules to produce a reaction with azido, resulting in a stable triazole linkage (Figure 2.1) [41]. Tan *et al.* successfully synthesized OB functionalized chitosan (CS–OB) and azido functionalized hyaluronan (HA–N_3) for hydrogel preparation via OB-azide [3+2] cycloaddition. The authors compared the DNA content of the human adipose-derived stem cells (hASCs), *in vitro* cell viability, and *in situ* biocompatibility in the control copper-catalyzed hydrogels to that of metal-free click hydrogels. The DNA content in the copper-catalyzed hydrogel progressively decreased after encapsulation with a significant reduction after 14 and 21 days of culture. As for the metal-free click hydrogel, there was no significant change of DNA quantity in the initial 7 days of culture; however, the DNA content significantly increased after 14 and 21 days of culture. In the metal-free hydrogel, most of the encapsulated hASCs survived after 21 days of culture and retained regular spherical morphologies while only few live cells were observed in the copper-catalyzed hydrogel after 21 days of incubation (Figure 2.2). Additionally, the metal-free click hydrogel showed promising biocompatibility in the preliminary murine *in situ* studies [14].

Truong *et al.* prepared a hydrogel based on water-soluble azide-functionalized chitosan (CS–N_3) and propiolic acid ester-functional PEG using [3+2] cycloaddition copper-free click chemistry. The resultant hydrogels formed within 5–60 minutes at physiological temperature due to 1, 3-dipolar cycloaddition of azides (CS–N_3) with electron-deficient alkynes (3-arm PEG containing an activated ester alkyne group) and gave rise to mechanically robust materials. Of great significance, was the ability of the hydrogels to support human bone marrow mesenchymal stem cell (hMSC) attachment and proliferation with zero toxicity to the encapsulated cells [15].

2.3 THIOL-ENE CLICK REACTION

Typically, a thiol-ene click chemistry reaction refers to the reaction of thiol-containing compounds with alkenes, or "-enes." Interest in thiol-ene click chemistry for hydrogel design has emerged from several attributes: (i) high efficiency under mild conditions

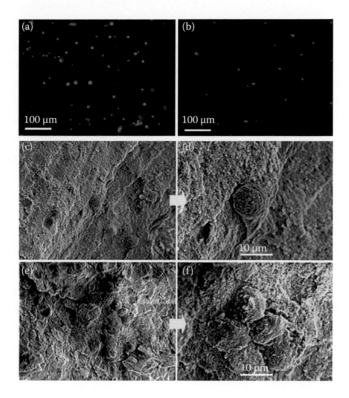

FIGURE 2.2 Confocal laser scanning microscopy images showing human adipose-derived stem cells (hASCs) encapsulated in the metal-free (a) and copper-catalyzed (b) hydrogels after 21 days of culture. The live cells were stained with Cell Tracker Orange CMRA and all cell nuclei were stained with Hoechst 33342. Scanning electron microscopy images show the morphology of encapsulated ASCs after 7 days (c, d) and 21 days (e, f) of culture. Adapted from Fan *et al.* [14], with permission from Elsevier.

(*in situ*, water, and buffers) and biocompatibility with cells and other biological molecules [12], (ii) well-defined and well-characterized reaction mechanisms and products proceeding by either radically mediated thiol-ene reactions or thiol-Michael-type reactions, and (iii) ease of introduction of thiols and alkenes to macromolecules for hydrogel synthesis compared to the process of introducing other functional groups (*in situ*, strained cyclooctynes) [42, 43].

2.3.1 Thiol-ene Photo Click Reaction

In radically mediated thiol-ene chemistry, an initiator is needed to produce radicals, which begin the reaction between thiols and select alkene functional groups. Radical generation can be achieved using thermal, oxidation-reduction, or photochemical processes based on initiator selection. Unlike the traditional free radical chain polymerization (*in situ*, (meth)acrylates), radically mediated thiol-ene reactions are relatively oxygen-insensitive. The photochemical processes are most widely utilized and are particularly attractive for designing thiol-ene hydrogels for biomedical applications as they afford spatiotemporal control of the polymerization by regulating the application of light [42–44].

2.3.1.1 Thiol-(Meth)Acrylate Photo Click

The properties of thiol-(meth)acrylate photo click hydrogels can be tuned by changing light intensities, light exposure time, PEG functionality (4-arm vs. 2-arm), and the polymer weight percentage [4]. However, ultraviolet (UV) light may compromise cytocompatibility because of the production of cytotoxic free radicals, which damage cellular proteins and DNA. Also, it has been shown that certain cell types (osteoblasts and corneal epithelial cells) are very sensitive to UV light [45]. To reduce phototoxicity, Fu *et al.* prepared numerous heparin-based hydrogels that can be cured *in situ* with visible light. This heparin-based hydrogel used eosin Y as a photoinitiator and triethanolamine as an electron donor to initiate a reaction of thiolated-heparin with acrylate-terminated PEG. Formulations and irradiation conditions are presented for control of heparin content (1.6%–3.3% w/v), storage modulus (100–10,000 Pa), and gelation time (30–600 seconds). In particular, irradiation conditions that achieve gelation in 150 seconds are compatible with the stringent light exposure limits of the retina, which affords a wide safety margin for use with other tissues. Using a 4-arm PEG instead of a linear PEG (2-arm PEG) led to a faster gelation time and higher modulus. Encapsulation of 3T3 fibroblasts in the hydrogel produced more than 96% viability for all conditions examined. *In vitro* characterization of the epidermal growth factor released from the hydrogel confirmed that the growth factor remained bioactive [16].

2.3.1.2 Thiol-Norbornene Photo Click

A thiol-norbornene photo click reaction refers to orthogonal reactions between multifunctional norbornene-modified macromers and sulfhydryl-containing linkers mediated by light. Hydrogels prepared by thiol-norbornene photo click have diverse material systems for tissue engineering applications because of the following advantages: (i) the gelation of thiol-norbornene hydrogels can be initiated by either long-wave UV light or visible light without additional co-initiators or co-monomers; (ii) unlike a thiol-(meth)acrylate photo click reaction, there is no chain growth polymerization of acrylate in a thiol-norbornene reaction [46]; (iii) the cross-linking and degradation behaviors of these hydrogels are controlled through material selections, whereas the biophysical and biochemical properties of the gels can be easily and independently tuned because of the orthogonal reactivity between norbornene and thiol moieties.

The Anseth group cross-linked norbornene-functionalized PEG with cysteine-containing peptides via thiol-norbornene photo click [17]. The resulting hydrogels promoted neuronal survival and axon outgrowth through cell-extracellular matrix interactions, such as those between the laminin-derived peptide YIGSR (Tyr–Ile–Gly–Ser–Arg) and its integrin, and allowed the neurons to remodel their extracellular environment through matrix metalloproteinase (MMP)-mediated polymer network degradation. This work demonstrated the development of a 3D platform for the culture of both aggregated and single mammalian motor nerve cells that not only permit cell survival over more than a week of culture but also allow for the robust extension of motor axons [17]. The Anseth group also encapsulated hMSCs in thiol-norbornene hydrogels with different degrees of MMP-sensitivity and studied the impact of matrix compositions on osteogenic, adipogenic, and chondrogenic differentiation of hMSCs in 3D [18]. Lin *et al.* prepared PEG hydrogels by the thiol-norbornene photo click, which exhibited a high degree of tunability in network cross-linking and degradation. The gelation rate of reaction had been controlled by varying the light intensity, wavelength, and photoinitiator concentrations. Compared to Michael-type addition hydrogels (Section 3.2) [46], thiol-norbornene photo click hydrogels formed with a shorter gelation time and a higher degree of cross-linking. They were hydrolytically degradable and followed a bulk degradation mechanism when base-catalyzed [47].

Although thiol-ene photo click reactions provide a promising platform for the development of hydrogels with acceptable physical and chemical properties, their clinical use is limited by the cytocompatibility and the depth of light penetration. While hydrogels may be formed *in situ* during surgical procedures without a need for light penetration, the formation of hydrogels by irradiation through the tissues is currently limited to superficial depths by the scattering of light by the tissues (*in situ*, penetration depths of ~0.5 mm at 365–500 nm through the skin) [48, 49].

2.3.2 Thiol-Michael-Type Click

A thiol-Michael-type addition reaction, or the conjugate addition of thiols or thiolate anions to electron-deficient C=C bonds with or without the help of a basic catalyst, has garnered significant attention, primarily due to its facile, powerful nature. Typical electron-deficient -enes in thiol-Michael-type addition reactions consist of acrylates, methacrylates, vinyl sulfones, and maleimides (Figure 2.1), as well as other electron-deficient propiolates and -ynes, such as -ynones. Typically, the more electron-deficient the C=C bond, the more susceptible it is to a Michael-type addition reaction. Therefore, the order of reactivity in terms of the C=C bond reactivity is as follows: maleimides > vinyl sulfones > acrylate & acrylamides > methacrylates [42].

2.3.2.1 Thiol-(Meth)Acrylate Michael Reaction

Acryloyl groups (H$_2$C=CH–C(=O)–) contain double bonds that are electron poor in nature and react with thiols to form stable thioether linkages (Figure 2.1) under alkaline conditions or in the presence of free radicals [50]. Recently, we developed a novel biomimetic hydrogel system as a tunable stem cell niche through the combination of thiolated HA (HA-SH) and thiolated CS (CS-SH) cross-linked with PEG-diacrylate (PEG-DA). The combination of HA and CS offers a cell-friendly microenvironment found in native tissues, whereas the selection of PEG is based on its established biocompatibility and chemical versatility. We showed the efficient control of various hydrogel properties by simply varying the PEG molecular weight. We also demonstrated that the composite hydrogels could support 3D encapsulation of hMSCs with high viability as well as tunable cell-hydrogel interactions by varying the properties of hydrogels. The ability to precisely control hydrogel properties paves the way for further optimization of cellular responses to promote *in situ* tissue regeneration [51].

2.3.2.2 Thiol-Vinyl Sulfone Michael Reaction

Vinyl sulfones (VS) are electron-poor alkenes that react with thiols in slightly alkaline conditions (*in situ*, pH ~8) to give stable β-thiosulfonyl linkages, known as thioether bonds (Figure 2.1). VS groups are generally stable for extended periods under aqueous conditions near neutral pH.

The Feijen group cross-linked thiolated HA (HA-SH) and PEG vinyl sulfone (PEG-VS) macromers via Michael-type additions to form hydrogels under physiological conditions. Gelation times, enzymatic degradation, and the storage modulus depended on the molecular weights of macromers, degree of substitution of HA-SH, and total polymer concentration [52]. The hydrogels showed good biocompatibility and high potential for cartilage regeneration, as demonstrated from accumulated collagen II, chondroitin sulfate, and glycosaminoglycans after culturing chondrocytes in these hydrogels for 21 days [52]. Shikanov *et al.* prepared bioactive PEG hydrogels via a Michael-type addition between GCGYGRGDSPG-modified multiarm VS functional PEG and a trifunctional protease sensitive cross-linking peptide. Bioactive modification influenced the mechanical properties of multiarm PEG gels, such as storage modulus and swelling. These changes were dependent on PEG functionality (4-arm vs. 8-arm) and PEG weight percentages, which were directly related to the concentration of elastically active chains and the overall amount of binding sites. Overall, the 8-arm PEG allowed a greater degree of modification and its macroscopic properties and cross-linking kinetics were less affected by the act of modification or quenching compared to the 4-arm PEG [22].

2.3.2.3 Thiol-Maleimide Michael Reaction

Maleimides (MAL) are electron-poor alkenes and readily react with thiols by Michael-type additions to form succinimide thioether linkages (Figure 2.1). Thiol-maleimide reactions offer several advantages: (i) thiol-maleimide reactions could react at neutral pH with high selectivity; (ii) compared with other types of alkenes, maleimide generally react faster with thiol under physiological conditions; and (iii) under reducing conditions for controlled degradation and release applications, the thiol-maleimide linkage formed with aryl thiols can undergo retro-Michael-type reactions. Nevertheless, it is necessary to note that in aqueous conditions, maleimide groups undergo ring hydrolysis and then would yield maleamic acid, which is not reactive with thiols. However, maleimide ring hydrolysis after the hydrogel formation will not significantly change the properties of an existing hydrogel; ring hydrolysis in the precursor solution before hydrogel preparation can significantly increase network defects, which typically increase mesh size and reduce network retention of loaded therapeutics, and consecutively can affect the release characteristics. Furthermore, thorough purification of maleimide-functionalized macromers after synthesis is needed because unreacted small-molecule maleimides can be cytotoxic [53]. Therefore, considerable caution must be applied in handling and implementing any reactions that utilize maleimides, which are known neurotoxins [42].

Phelps *et al.* prepared 4-arm PEG-maleimide (PEG-4MAL) hydrogels by incorporating cell adhesive ligands via Michael-type additions and compared it to a 4-arm PEG-acrylate (PEG-4A), a 4-arm PEG-4VS, and a UV photo-cross-linked PEG-DA. PEG-4MAL exhibits faster reaction kinetics and a tighter network structure than PEG-4A or PEG-4VS. Additionally, the PEG-4MAL cross-linking reaction requires two orders of magnitude less triethyl amine than either PEG-4A or PEG-4VS. Furthermore, PEG-4MAL hydrogels require a lower polymer weight percentage and possess a wider range of Young's moduli than hydrogels based on PEG-DA, PEG-4A, and PEG-4VS. These lower polymer weight percentage PEG-4MAL networks promoted increased spreading of encapsulated cells that could not be recapitulated in PEG-DA, PEG-4A, or PEG-4VS hydrogels. PEG-4MAL hydrogels had significantly faster gelation times of 1–5 minutes depending on the weight percentage and held a strong potential for clinical use with *in situ* gelation [23]. Darling *et al.* also proved that the thiolate addition to the PEG maleimide bond is a faster and more efficient reaction than the thiolate addition to the PEG acrylate bond. However, the fast gelation kinetics of the thiol-maleimide reaction lead to inefficient mixing, heterogeneous gelation, and inconsistent cell responses to the hydrogel in these regions of high and low cross-linking. The gelation rate of thiol-maleimide cross-linked hydrogels can be slowed with the addition of either zinc chloride or a metalloproteinase-sensitive peptide tag sequence to overcome the cellular response variability between batches [26].

Thiol-ene click reactions suffer from several limitations despite their broad applications. Thiol-functionalized macromers can react with each other to form disulfide linkages, making them inaccessible for a subsequent reaction with alkenes and posing a challenge in the consistent formation of thiol-ene hydrogels. Additionally, thiols on macromers can react with various functional groups that are present on biologics (i.e., off-target reactions leading to oxidation of cysteine residues on proteins) [53]. Thiol-disulfide oxidoreduction of cell surface proteins plays a role in regulating critical cellular functions, such as adhesion and proliferation [54]; thus, a blank hydrogel canvas without thiols allows more control over cellular behavior.

2.4 DIELS–ALDER REACTIONS

The Diels–Alder (DA) reaction is a highly selective [4+2] cycloaddition between a diene and a dienophile that is greatly accelerated in water [55]. Furthermore, the DA is free from side reactions and by-products, allows for the formation and functionalization of numerous molecules without any catalysts or initiators, and provides an extremely selective reaction.

Nimmo *et al.* were the first to design a simple one-step, aqueous-based cross-linking system to synthesize a HA hydrogel through a DA reaction of furan-modified HA (HA-furan) with dimaleimide PEG for tissue engineering applications. However, the reaction conditions involved a 100 mM 2-(*N*-morpholino)-ethanesulfonic acid (MES) buffer at pH 5.5, which is not suitable for 3D cellular encapsulation (reaction temperature and time were not reported) [56]. Both the mechanical and degradation properties of these HA/PEG hydrogels can be tuned via controlling the furan-to-maleimide molar ratio or polymer weight percentages. The HA/PEG hydrogels had an elastic modulus ranging from 275 to 680 Pa (similar to that of the central nervous system tissue) and possessed minimal swelling and complete degradation over time. Human epithelial cells plated on top of the hydrogel showed cellular attachment within 24 hours, interacted with the hydrogels after 14 days of culture *in vitro*, and exhibited high viability [56]. Biomolecules, such as proteins, were photopatterned into these HA-furan/PEG DA hydrogels by two-photon laser processing, resulting in spatially defined growth factor gradients to direct cell function [30]. Tan *et al.* also prepared an HA-based hydrogel as a therapeutically effective platform for adipose tissue engineering by cross-linking the HA-furan and the maleimide-modified HA derivative [33, 34]. In another study, Yu *et al.* prepared interpenetrating HA/gelatin/CS biomimetic hydrogels. This was done by cross-linking HA-furan and furan-functionalized gelatin (G-furan) via dimaleimide PEG and then further cross-linking via CS through a 1-ethyl-3-(-3-dimethylaminopropyl) carbodiimide hydrochloride (EDC)/N-hydroxysuccinimide (NHS) reaction [35]. Other investigations of similar chemistry included the synthesis of HA hydrogels [57] and hydroxypropyl methylcellulose-based hydrogels [58]. Although these DA hydrogels have efficient chemical bonding and tunable mechanical properties, their application in cell encapsulation and in biologically relevant systems was limited by the long gelation time and non-injectable properties.

Generally, a gelation time of several hours or days at room temperature is necessary for DA-formed hydrogels. To overcome this obstacle of the DA-formed hydrogels, Yu *et al.* prepared a novel biological hydrogel from HA and PEG using DA click chemistry. By simply tuning the furyl-to-maleimide molar ratio and the substitution degree of the furyl group, the value of the compressive modulus was controlled from 4.86 ± 0.42 to 75.90 ± 5.43 kPa, and the gelation time could be tuned from 412 to 51 minutes at 37°C. Moreover, the DA-formed hydrogel was utilized to investigate the cell encapsulation viability and the influence of gelation time on encapsulated cell survival. The results showed that a gelation time of about 1 hour was suitable for cell viability, proliferation, and chondrogenesis. The gene expression levels of the chondrogenesis markers collagen II and aggrecan were significantly upregulated both with and without growth factor TGF-β3. Additionally, as shown in Figure 2.3, the HA/PEG hydrogel showed outstanding load-bearing and shape recovery properties even after 2,000 loading cycles, mimicking the mechanical properties and behavior of articular cartilage [28].

Efforts have also been made to combine a DA reaction with other cross-linker methods to facilitate gelation. For example, an injectable hyaluronic acid/PEG (HA/PEG) hydrogel was successfully fabricated by performing two cross-linking processes: first, enzymatic cross-linking, and second, DA click chemistry. The enzymatic cross-linking resulted in gelation of HA/PEG after 5 minutes, leading to the formation of an injectable material while the DA click reaction cross-linking produced a hydrogel with outstanding shape memory and anti-fatigue properties. After 10 cycles of a loading and unloading test, the hydrogel still could be loaded by 80 kPa for 1 minute, and the corresponding deformation could be completely recovered in 1 minute after unloading. The chondrogenic ATDC-5 cells were encapsulated into the hydrogel bulk *in situ* and showed high metabolic viability and proliferation [29].

Another reaction related to the DA reaction, called the retro-DA (rDA), results from the decomposition of certain DA (or hDA) products, which could be attributed to the degradation of DA hydrogels [59]. Kirchhof *et al.* investigated cross-linking and degradation mechanism of DA hydrogels that were cross-linked by furyl and maleimide functionalized PEG [60]. The maleimide groups were subject to ring-opening hydrolysis at a level above pH 5.5, with pH and temperature being the main influencing factors, which directly affects the cross-linking and degradation behavior of DA hydrogels. Cross-linking is best performed in slightly acidic solutions (e.g., at pH 5.5) to ensure high degrees of conversion.

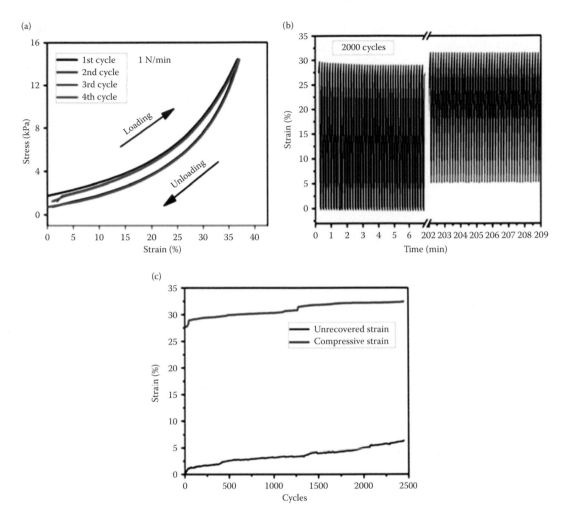

FIGURE 2.3 (a) Four successive hydrogel loading–unloading cycles. The ramp force loading rate and unloading rates were 1 and −1 N min⁻¹. (b) Strain recovery of the hydrogels <2,000 cycles of force loading and unloading. (Each loading stress was kept at 20 kPa.) (c) The variation tendency of the hydrogel compressive strain and unrecovered strain after 2,500 loading cycles. Reproduced from Yan *et al.* [37], with permission from the Royal Society of Chemistry.

Furthermore, cross-linking above room temperature (e.g., at 37°C) resulted in a faster gelation process. The complex shear modulus was also dependent on the concentration, branching factor, and molecular weight of the macromonomer. The swelling and degradation of hydrogels were influenced by the same parameters. With increasing pH and temperature, the degradation time was reduced from 98 days (pH 7.4, 20°C) to 2 days (pH 7.4, 50°C); no degradation was observed at levels of pH 3.0 and 5.5. The molecular modeling studies of the DA and rDA moieties revealed that hydrogel degradation occurred by an rDA reaction followed by OH⁻-catalyzed ring-opening hydrolysis of maleimide groups to unreactive maleamic acid derivatives. The removal of maleimide groups from the DA/rDA equilibrium by ring-opening hydrolysis increased the rate of the rDA reaction, which avoided the need for high temperatures to incite the rDA reaction, thus allowing the synthesis of bio-materials that readily degrade at physiological conditions [32, 60].

Recently, an inverse electron demand Diels–Alder (iEDDA) reaction, a more intriguing and promising type of DA reaction, was considered as a potential click reaction almost simultaneously in 2008 by Devaraj et al. [61] and others. Opposed to normal electron demand DA reactions, the tetrazine dienes are electron deficient while the dienophiles that are electron-rich are preferred in the iEDDA reaction [59]. Truong *et al.* reported the simultaneous application of nucleophilic thiol-yne and iEDDA additions to independently create two interpenetrating networks in a simple one-step procedure. The resultant hydro-gels display compressive stresses of 14–15 MPa at 98% compression without fracture or hysteresis on repeated load. The hydrogel networks can be spatially and temporally post functionalized via radical thiylation and/or iEDDA addition to residual functional groups within the network. Furthermore, gelation occurs rapidly under physiological conditions, thus enabling encapsulation of human cells [62].

2.5 ALDEHYDE-HYDRAZIDE AND OXIME CLICK REACTIONS

The aldehyde-hydrazide reaction (also referred to Schiff base reaction) has become an attractive approach for bioconjugation [63] because the amino groups efficiently and orthogonally form imine bonds with aldehyde groups without any external stimulus and extraneous reagents under physiological conditions. Another advantage of the aldehyde-hydrazide reaction is that the aldehyde groups contained in hydrogel further promote good integration of the hydrogel to the surrounding tissues [64].

Various hydrogels have been fabricated from PEG or the polysaccharide adipic acid dihydrazide (ADH) and aldehyde derivatives via aldehyde-hydrazide reaction. Recently, Yan *et al.* fabricated injectable hydrogels by self-cross-linking of hydrazide-modified poly (L-glutamic acid) and aldehyde-modified alginate (ALG-CHO). The gelation time, equilibrium swelling, degradation rate, microscopic morphology, and rheological properties could be adjusted by varying the solid content of the hydrogels and oxidation degree of ALG-CHO. The encapsulation of rabbit chondrocytes within hydrogels showed viability of the entrapped cells and good biocompatibility of the injectable hydrogels. A preliminary study exhibited injectability and rapid *in situ* gel formation, as well as cell ingrowth and ectopic chondrogenesis [37]. More recently, Cao, Yu *et al.* synthesized an injectable hydrogel via *in situ* cross-linking of glycol chitosan (GC) and multi-benzaldehyde functionalized PEG analogues, poly(ethylene oxide-*co*-glycidol)-CHO, for cartilage tissue engineering [36]. The gelation time, water uptake, mechanical properties, and network morphology of the GC/(poly(EO-*co*-Gly) hydrogels were well modulated by varying the concentration of poly(EO-*co*-Gly)-CHO. Both *in vitro* and *in situ* testing confirmed the degradation of GC/poly(EO-*co*-Gly) hydrogels, and the lifetime of injected hydrogels *in situ* was greater than 3 months (Figure 2.4). Chondrocytes encapsulated in GC/poly(EO-*co*-Gly) hydrogels maintained a high viability and a round cell morphology after 14 days of 3D culture. The maintenance of the chondrocyte phenotype was also confirmed by examining the characteristic gene expression [36]. Yu, Chen *et al.* prepared a multifunctional hydrogel via the integration of DA click chemistry and an acylhydrazone bond [38]. The DA reaction

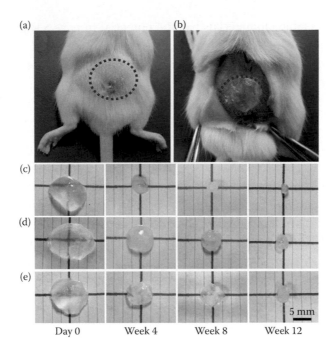

FIGURE 2.4 Global view after subcutaneous injection of the GC/poly(EO-*co*-Gly) hydrogel containing 0.5 wt% poly(EO-*co*-Gly)-CHO and 1.5 wt% GC into an Imprinting Control Region (ICR) mouse (a), and subsequently, dissection 30 minutes post injection (b). The dashed circles indicate the presence of *in situ* formed hydrogels. (c–e) Photographs of the remaining hydrogels containing the indicated concentrations of poly(EO-*co*-Gly)-CHO: (c) 0.25 wt%, (d) 0.5 wt% and (e) 2.0 wt% removed from ICR mice after 0–12 weeks. The final concentration of GC in the hydrogels was fixed at 1.5 wt%. Reproduced from Cao *et al.* [36], with permission from the Royal Society of Chemistry.

maintained the hydrogel structural integrity and mechanical strength in a physiological environment, while the dynamic covalent acylhydrazone bond resulted in self-healing properties and controlled the on/off switch of network cross-link density. At the same time, integration of the hydrogel to the surrounding tissues was achieved by an aldehyde-hydrazide reaction. This type of hydrogel has good structural integrity, autonomous self-healing, and tissue-adhesive properties and simultaneously will have good applications in tissue engineering and the tissue repair field [38].

Oxime click chemistry, the formation of an oxime bond by a reaction between an aminooxy group and an aldehyde or ketone, has emerged as a robust strategy in areas such as bioconjugation (Table 2.1) [65]. Grover, Christman *et al.* prepared an injectable hydrogel utilizing oxime cross-linking. Tunable *in vitro* gelation was achieved by altering the pH with a bioinert-PEG system, as well as with oxidized hyaluronic acid and alginate [39]. Oxime chemistry allowed for these materials to be injected multiple times through a catheter *in vitro* over the course of hours while at 37°C, thus mimicking the *in situ* situation. The PEG and polysaccharide systems form gels within 20 minutes after injection into the subcutaneous space. The PEG-oxime system was capable of rapid gelation on injection into the myocardial tissue. Overall, the resulting data demonstrated that oxime cross-linking of injectable biomaterials has the potential to pave a way for more difficult, minimally invasive delivery routes that require a material to be held at body temperature for extended periods of time, yet gel quickly once it enters the tissue (i.e., catheter-based delivery in the heart) [39].

2.6 CONCLUSIONS

In summary, click reactions provide powerful and versatile tools for the rational design of novel functional hydrogels for regenerative engineering applications. The high coupling efficiency and specificity, bioorthogonality, and mild reaction conditions of click chemistry impart hydrogels with unique and tunable properties. In particular, click chemistry enables the optimization of new hydrogel scaffolds for directing stem cell differentiation and/or guiding cell attachment and growth. The click hydrogels, especially the injectable hydrogels, have also demonstrated great translational potential as effective carriers for various cells, proteins, peptides, and therapeutics. Future work on understanding and regulating cell–biomaterial interactions using hydrogel-based cell niches will foster the successful translation of regenerative engineering of complex tissue interfaces and tissue systems.

ACKNOWLEDGMENTS

Funding support from NIH R03AR068108, Showalter Trust, Purdue Research Foundation, and Purdue Start-up Package is greatly appreciated.

REFERENCES

1. C.T. Laurencin, Y. Khan, Regenerative engineering, *Science Translational Medicine* 4(160) (2012) 160ed9–160ed9.
2. M. Deng, R. James, C.T. Laurencin, S.G. Kumbar, Nanostructured polymeric scaffolds for orthopaedic regenerative engineering, *IEEE Transactions on NanoBioscience* 11(1) (2012) 3–14.
3. H.C. Kolb, M.G. Finn, K.B. Sharpless, Click chemistry: Diverse chemical function from a few good reactions, *Angewandte Chemie-International Edition* 40(11) (2001) 2004–2021.
4. W. Xi, T.F. Scott, C.J. Kloxin, C.N. Bowman, Click chemistry in materials science, *Advanced Functional Materials* 24(18) (2014) 2572–2590.
5. D.A. Ossipov, J. Hilborn, Poly (vinyl alcohol)-based hydrogels formed by "click chemistry," *Macromolecules* 39(5) (2006) 1709–1718.
6. S.Q. Liu, P.L. Rachel Ee, C.Y. Ke, J.L. Hedrick, Y.Y. Yang, Biodegradable poly(ethylene glycol)–peptide hydrogels with well-defined structure and properties for cell delivery, *Biomaterials* 30(8) (2009) 1453–1461.
7. M. van Dijk, C.F. van Nostrum, W.E. Hennink, D.T.S. Rijkers, R.M.J. Liskamp, Synthesis and characterization of enzymatically biodegradable PEG and peptide-based hydrogels prepared by click chemistry, *Biomacromolecules* 11(6) (2010) 1608–1614.
8. R.T. Chen, S. Marchesan, R.A. Evans, K.E. Styan, G.K. Such, A. Postma, K.M. McLean, B.W. Muir, F. Caruso, Photoinitiated alkyne–azide click and radical cross-linking reactions for the patterning of PEG hydrogels, *Biomacromolecules* 13(3) (2012) 889–895.
9. A. Koschella, M. Hartlieb, T. Heinze, A "click-chemistry" approach to cellulose-based hydrogels, *Carbohydrate Polymers* 86(1) (2011) 154–161.

10. V. Crescenzi, L. Cornelio, C. Di Meo, S. Nardecchia, R. Lamanna, Novel hydrogels via click chemistry: Synthesis and potential biomedical applications, *Biomacromolecules* 8(6) (2007) 1844–1850.
11. X. Hu, D. Li, F. Zhou, C. Gao, Biological hydrogel synthesized from hyaluronic acid, gelatin and chondroitin sulfate by click chemistry, *Acta Biomaterialia* 7(4) (2011) 1618–1626.
12. A. Takahashi, Y. Suzuki, T. Suhara, K. Omichi, A. Shimizu, K. Hasegawa, N. Kokudo, S. Ohta, T. Ito, In situ cross-linkable hydrogel of hyaluronan produced via copper-free click chemistry, *Biomacromolecules* 14(10) (2013) 3581–3588.
13. H. Jiang, S. Qin, H. Dong, Q. Lei, X. Su, R. Zhuo, Z. Zhong, An injectable and fast-degradable poly(ethylene glycol) hydrogel fabricated via bioorthogonal strain-promoted azide–alkyne cycloaddition click chemistry, *Soft Matter* 11(30) (2015) 6029–6036.
14. M. Fan, Y. Ma, J. Mao, Z. Zhang, H. Tan, Cytocompatible in situ forming chitosan/hyaluronan hydrogels via a metal-free click chemistry for soft tissue engineering, *Acta Biomaterialia* 20 (2015) 60–68.
15. V.X. Truong, M.P. Ablett, H.T.J. Gilbert, J. Bowen, S.M. Richardson, J.A. Hoyland, A.P. Dove, In situ-forming robust chitosan-poly(ethylene glycol) hydrogels prepared by copper-free azide–alkyne click reaction for tissue engineering, *Biomaterials Science* 2(2) (2014) 167–175.
16. A. Fu, K. Gwon, M. Kim, G. Tae, J.A. Kornfield, Visible-light-initiated thiol–acrylate photopolymerization of heparin-based hydrogels, *Biomacromolecules* 16(2) (2015) 497–506.
17. D.D. McKinnon, A.M. Kloxin, K.S. Anseth, Synthetic hydrogel platform for three-dimensional culture of embryonic stem cell-derived motor neurons, *Biomaterials Science* 1(5) (2013) 460–469.
18. S.B. Anderson, C.C. Lin, D.V. Kuntzler, K.S. Anseth, The performance of human mesenchymal stem cells encapsulated in cell-degradable polymer-peptide hydrogels, *Biomaterials* 32(14) (2011) 3564–3574.
19. J.A. Benton, B.D. Fairbanks, K.S. Anseth, Characterization of valvular interstitial cell function in three dimensional matrix metalloproteinase degradable PEG hydrogels, *Biomaterials* 30(34) (2009) 6593–6603.
20. K.A. Kyburz, K.S. Anseth, Three-dimensional hMSC motility within peptide-functionalized PEG-based hydrogel of varying adhesivity and crosslinking density, *Acta Biomaterialia* 9(5) (2013) 6381–6392.
21. S. Ouasti, R. Donno, F. Cellesi, M.J. Sherratt, G. Terenghi, N. Tirelli, Network connectivity, mechanical properties and cell adhesion for hyaluronic acid/PEG hydrogels, *Biomaterials* 32(27) (2011) 6456–6470.
22. J. Kim, Y.P. Kong, S.M. Niedzielski, R.K. Singh, A.J. Putnam, A. Shikanov, Characterization of the crosslinking kinetics of multi-arm poly(ethylene glycol) hydrogels formed via Michael-type addition, *Soft Matter* 12(7) (2016) 2076–2085.
23. E.A. Phelps, N.O. Enemchukwu, V.F. Fiore, J.C. Sy, N. Murthy, T.A. Sulchek, T.H. Barker, A.J. García, Maleimide cross-linked bioactive PEG hydrogel exhibits improved reaction kinetics and cross-linking for cell encapsulation and in situ delivery, *Advanced Materials* 24(1) (2012) 64–70.
24. J. Kim, I.S. Kim, T.H. Cho, K.B. Lee, S.J. Hwang, G. Tae, I. Noh, S.H. Lee, Y. Park, K. Sun, Bone regeneration using hyaluronic acid-based hydrogel with bone morphogenic protein-2 and human mesenchymal stem cells, *Biomaterials* 28(10) (2007) 1830–1837.
25. R. Jin, L.M. Teixeira, A. Krouwels, P. Dijkstra, C. Van Blitterswijk, M. Karperien, J. Feijen, Synthesis and characterization of hyaluronic acid–poly (ethylene glycol) hydrogels via Michael addition: An injectable biomaterial for cartilage repair, *Acta Biomaterialia* 6(6) (2010) 1968–1977.
26. N.J. Darling, Y.-S. Hung, S. Sharma, T. Segura, Controlling the kinetics of thiol-maleimide Michael-type addition gelation kinetics for the generation of homogenous poly(ethylene glycol) hydrogels, *Biomaterials* 101 (2016) 199–206.

27. Z. Zeng, X.-m. Mo, C. He, Y. Morsi, H. El-Hamshary, M. El-Newehy, An in situ forming tissue adhesive based on poly (ethylene glycol)-dimethacrylate and thiolated chitosan through the Michael reaction, *Journal of Materials Chemistry B* 4(33) (2016) 5585–5592.

28. F. Yu, X. Cao, Y. Li, L. Zeng, J. Zhu, G. Wang, X. Chen, Diels–Alder crosslinked HA/PEG hydrogels with high elasticity and fatigue resistance for cell encapsulation and articular cartilage tissue repair, *Polymer Chemistry* 5(17) (2014) 5116–5123.

29. F. Yu, X. Cao, Y. Li, L. Zeng, B. Yuan, X. Chen, An injectable hyaluronic acid/PEG hydrogel for cartilage tissue engineering formed by integrating enzymatic crosslinking and Diels–Alder "click chemistry", *Polymer Chemistry* 5(3) (2014) 1082–1090.

30. S.C. Owen, S.A. Fisher, R.Y. Tam, C.M. Nimmo, M.S. Shoichet, Hyaluronic acid click hydrogels emulate the extracellular matrix, *Langmuir* 29(24) (2013) 7393–7400.

31. C.M. Nimmo, S.C. Owen, M.S. Shoichet, Diels–Alder click cross-linked hyaluronic acid hydrogels for tissue engineering, *Biomacromolecules* 12(3) (2011) 824–830.

32. S. Kirchhof, A. Strasser, H.-J. Wittmann, V. Messmann, N. Hammer, A.M. Goepferich, F.P. Brandl, New insights into the cross-linking and degradation mechanism of Diels–Alder hydrogels, *Journal of Materials Chemistry B* 3(3) (2015) 449–457.

33. M. Fan, Y. Ma, Z. Zhang, J. Mao, H. Tan, X. Hu, Biodegradable hyaluronic acid hydrogels to control release of dexamethasone through aqueous Diels–Alder chemistry for adipose tissue engineering, *Materials Science and Engineering: C* 56 (2015) 311–317.

34. Y. Jia, M. Fan, H. Chen, Y. Miao, L. Xing, B. Jiang, Q. Cheng, D. Liu, W. Bao, B. Qian, J. Wang, X. Xing, H. Tan, Z. Ling, Y. Chen, Magnetic hyaluronic acid nanospheres via aqueous Diels–Alder chemistry to deliver dexamethasone for adipose tissue engineering, *Journal of Colloid and Interface Science* 458 (2015) 293–299.

35. F. Yu, X. Cao, L. Zeng, Q. Zhang, X. Chen, An interpenetrating HA/G/CS biomimic hydrogel via Diels–Alder click chemistry for cartilage tissue engineering, *Carbohydrate Polymers* 97(1) (2013) 188–195.

36. L. Cao, B. Cao, C. Lu, G. Wang, L. Yu, J. Ding, An injectable hydrogel formed by in situ cross-linking of glycol chitosan and multi-benzaldehyde functionalized PEG analogues for cartilage tissue engineering, *Journal of Materials Chemistry B* 3(7) (2015) 1268–1280.

37. S. Yan, T. Wang, L. Feng, J. Zhu, K. Zhang, X. Chen, L. Cui, J. Yin, Injectable in situ selfcross-linking hydrogels based on poly(L-glutamic acid) and alginate for cartilage tissue engineering, *Biomacromolecules* 15(12) (2014) 4495–4508.

38. F. Yu, X. Cao, J. Du, G. Wang, X. Chen, Multifunctional hydrogel with good structure integrity, self-healing, and tissue-adhesive property formed by combining Diels–Alder click reaction and acylhydrazone bond, *ACS Applied Materials & Interfaces* 7(43) (2015) 24023-24031.

39. G.N. Grover, R.L. Braden, K.L. Christman, Oxime cross-linked injectable hydrogels for catheter delivery, *Advanced Materials (Deerfield Beach, Fla.)* 25(21) (2013) 2937–2942.

40. N.J. Agard, J.A. Prescher, C.R. Bertozzi, A strain-promoted [3 + 2] azide–alkyne cycloaddition for covalent modification of biomolecules in living systems, *Journal of the American Chemical Society* 126(46) (2004) 15046–15047.

41. S.S. van Berkel, A.J. Dirks, M.F. Debets, F.L. van Delft, J.J.L.M. Cornelissen, R.J.M. Nolte, F.P.J.T. Rutjes, Metal-free triazole formation as a tool for bioconjugation, *ChemBioChem* 8(13) (2007) 1504–1508.

42. D.P. Nair, M. Podgórski, S. Chatani, T. Gong, W. Xi, C.R. Fenoli, C.N. Bowman, The thiol-Michael addition click reaction: A powerful and widely used tool in materials chemistry, *Chemistry of Materials* 26(1) (2014) 724–744.

43. C.E. Hoyle, C.N. Bowman, Thiol–ene click chemistry, *Angewandte Chemie International Edition* 49(9) (2010) 1540–1573.

44. K.S. Anseth, H.-A. Klok, Click chemistry in biomaterials, nanomedicine, and drug delivery, *Biomacromolecules* 17(1) (2016) 1–3.

45. C.G. Williams, A.N. Malik, T.K. Kim, P.N. Manson, J.H. Elisseeff, Variable cytocompatibility of six cell lines with photoinitiators used for polymerizing hydrogels and cell encapsulation, *Biomaterials* 26(11) (2005) 1211–1218.

46. C.-C. Lin, C.S. Ki, H. Shih, Thiol–norbornene photo-click hydrogels for tissue engineering applications, *Journal of Applied Polymer Science* 132(8) (2015) 41563.

47. H. Shih, C.-C. Lin, Cross-linking and degradation of step-growth hydrogels formed by thiol–ene photoclick chemistry, *Biomacromolecules* 13(7) (2012) 2003–2012.

48. F.H. Mustafa, M.S. Jaafar, Comparison of wavelength-dependent penetration depths of lasers in different types of skin in photodynamic therapy, *Indian Journal of Physics* 87(3) (2013) 203–209.

49. E. Maverakis, Y. Miyamura, M.P. Bowen, G. Correa, Y. Ono, H. Goodarzi, Light, including ultraviolet, *Journal of Autoimmunity* 34(3) (2010) J247–J257.

50. P.M. Kharkar, M.S. Rehmann, K.M. Skeens, E. Maverakis, A.M. Kloxin, Thiol–ene click hydrogels for therapeutic delivery, *ACS Biomaterials Science & Engineering* 2(2) (2016) 165–179.

51. L. Kuang, C. Jiang, G.N. Gellert, N.P. Damayanti, J. Irudayaraj, M. Deng, Bio-inspired composite hydrogels for musculoskeletal regenerative engineering, 10th World Biomaterials Congress, Frontiers in Bioengineering and Biotechnology, Montreal, May 17–22, 2016.

52. R. Jin, L.S. Moreira Teixeira, A. Krouwels, P.J. Dijkstra, C.A. van Blitterswijk, M. Karperien, J. Feijen, Synthesis and characterization of hyaluronic acid–poly(ethylene glycol) hydrogels via Michael addition: An injectable biomaterial for cartilage repair, *Acta Biomaterialia* 6(6) (2010) 1968–1977.

53. S. Chatani, D.P. Nair, C.N. Bowman, Relative reactivity and selectivity of vinyl sulfones and acrylates towards the thiol-Michael addition reaction and polymerization, *Polymer Chemistry* 4(4) (2013) 1048–1055.

54. J. Skalska, P.S. Brookes, S.M. Nadtochiy, S.P. Hilchey, C.T. Jordan, M.L. Guzman, S.B. Maggirwar, M.M. Briehl, S.H. Bernstein, Modulation of cell surface protein free thiols: A potential novel mechanism of action of the sesquiterpene lactone parthenolide, *PLoS One* 4(12) (2009) e8115.

55. S. Otto, J.B. Engberts, Hydrophobic interactions and chemical reactivity, *Organic & Biomolecular Chemistry* 1(16) (2003) 2809–2820.

56. C.M. Nimmo, S.C. Owen, M.S. Shoichet, Diels–Alder click cross-linked hyaluronic acid hydrogels for tissue engineering, *Biomacromolecules* 12(3) (2011) 824–830.

57. H. Tan, J.P. Rubin, K.G. Marra, Direct synthesis of biodegradable polysaccharide derivative hydrogels through aqueous Diels–Alder chemistry, *Macromolecular Rapid Communications* 32(12) (2011) 905–911.

58. G.-F. Wang, H.-J. Chu, H.-L. Wei, X.-Q. Liu, Z.-X. Zhao, J. Zhu, Click synthesis by Diels–Alder reaction and characterisation of hydroxypropyl methylcellulose-based hydrogels, *Chemical Papers* 68(10) (2014) 1390–1399.

59. L. Kuang, D.A. Fernandes, M. O'Halloran, W. Zheng, Y. Jiang, V. Ladizhansky, L.S. Brown, H. Liang, "Frozen" block copolymer nanomembranes with light-driven proton pumping performance, *ACS Nano* 8(1) (2014) 537–545.

60. S. Kirchhof, F.P. Brandl, N. Hammer, A.M. Goepferich, Investigation of the Diels–Alder reaction as a cross-linking mechanism for degradable poly(ethylene glycol) based hydrogels, *Journal of Materials Chemistry B* 1(37) (2013) 4855–4864.

61. N.K. Devaraj, R. Weissleder, S.A. Hilderbrand, Tetrazine-based cycloadditions: Application to pretargeted live cell imaging, *Bioconjugate Chemistry* 19(12) (2008) 2297–2299.

62. V.X. Truong, M.P. Ablett, S.M. Richardson, J.A. Hoyland, A.P. Dove, Simultaneous orthogonal dual-click approach to tough, in-situ-forming hydrogels for cell encapsulation, *Journal of the American Chemical Society* 137(4) (2015) 1618–1622.

63. D. Hua, J. Jiang, L. Kuang, J. Jiang, W. Zheng, H. Liang, Smart chitosan-based stimuli-responsive nanocarriers for the controlled delivery of hydrophobic pharmaceuticals, *Macromolecules* 44(6) (2011) 1298–1302.

64. D.-A. Wang, S. Varghese, B. Sharma, I. Strehin, S. Fermanian, J. Gorham, D.H. Fairbrother, B. Cascio, J.H. Elisseeff, Multifunctional chondroitin sulphate for cartilage tissue-biomaterial integration, *Nature Materials* 6(5) (2007) 385–392.

65. S. Ulrich, D. Boturyn, A. Marra, O. Renaudet, P. Dumy, Oxime ligation: A chemoselective click-type reaction for accessing multifunctional biomolecular constructs, *Chemistry: A European Journal* 20(1) (2014) 34–41.

CHAPTER 3

Bioactive Ceramics and Metals for Regenerative Engineering

Changchun Zhou, Xiangfeng Li, Junqiu Cheng, Hongsong Fan, and Xingdong Zhang

Sichuan University

CONTENTS

Regenerative engineering begins a new era for repairing damaged tissues or organs with the aim of creating living, functional tissue that has the ability to replace dysfunctional tissues or organs. While integrating the biological aspects of tissue regeneration via stem cells, factors, and cytokines, regenerative engineering requires the materials not only to be bioactive but also to stimulate specific biofunctions and cellular responses at the molecular level [1] and, thus, initiate tissue regeneration.

Among the bioactive materials applied in the clinic, bioactive ceramics and metals, as well as their composites, have always played important roles. This chapter will review related up-to-date and ongoing work in this area.

3.1 BIOACTIVE CERAMICS

3.1.1 Bioactive Ceramics and Their Challenges

Bioceramics are ceramic materials that have been specially developed for repairing hurt or damaged hard tissues, such as bone and teeth [2]. Most of the existing bioceramics are biocompatible, and some of them are bioactive with good bone bonding capability and have been applied successfully in the clinic [3–5]. The challenges for bioceramics mainly lie in the following three areas:

First, the brittleness and low resistance to fatigue of bioactive ceramics limit their application to bone defect filling. Table 3.1 shows the comparison between natural bone and several typical bioactive ceramics. Many efforts have been made to enhance the mechanical properties of ceramics. One of the widely applied methods is to create a composite using a polymer, either natural or synthetic [6–9], which is more flexible but softer than bioceramics. Normally, these composites show improved mechanical properties with good biological performances still being maintained. Another promising method is to develop nano-ceramic scaffolds. Nano-materials have more strength and toughness than conventional materials, and considerable research has demonstrated the improved mechanical strength as well as bioactivity. For example, hydroxyapatite (HA) nano-ceramics prepared by selective laser sintering showed outstanding mechanical properties and bioactivity which can induce bone regeneration [10].

Second, an important challenge for bioceramics is to be biodegradable with their degradation kinetics matching the living tissue formation, which is usually slower [20]. The ideal implants for regenerative engineering need to work as primary scaffolds and then degrade gradually and finally be replaced by the new tissue. Generally, the degradation rate of a

TABLE 3.1 Comparison between Natural Bone and Typical Bioactive Ceramics

Materials		Compression (MPa)	Flexure (MPa)	Elastic Modulus (GPa)
Natural bone [11, 12]	Compact	131–224	78.8–151	13.7
	Cancellous	3–20	3–20	1.5
Calcium-phosphate based ceramics [13, 14]	Dense	300–500	60–120	40–90
	Porous (≥50%)	<30	<20	<2
Silicate-based ceramics [15–17]	Dense	200–400	50–100	30–100
	Porous (≥50%)	<20	<20	<2
Polymer-ceramic composites [18, 19]	–	5–100	10–200	1–20

ceramic could be adjusted partly by varying the phase composition [4, 21]. For example, a composite mixture consisting of poorly soluble HA and highly soluble beta-tricalcium phosphate (β-TCP) with different phase ratios is considered to be able to achieve an optimal degradability [3, 22, 23]. Another efficient approach for adjusting the degradation rate of bioceramics is to be combined with a degradable polymer [7, 24, 25].

Finally, to date, there still remain several problems that bioactive ceramics must overcome, such as the toxicity of the degradation products, the complexity of the fabrication process, as well as the unsatisfied mechanical strength for load-bearing repair. The most effective way may be the fast and massive tissue formation within the scaffolds, which could lead to tissue regeneration and thus rebuild its biofunction. Therefore, to optimize and improve the bioactivity to induce tissue regeneration have always been the direction for research and development of bioactive ceramics [4, 26].

3.1.2 Bioactive Ceramics with Osteoinductivity for Regenerative Engineering

The first report of "osteoinduction" came from the work of Urist et al. who found the osteoinduction of BMP [27]. However, the discovery of osteoinduction of calcium phosphate (Ca-P) bioceramics highlighted the potential to explore a new generation of biomaterials. Ca-P osteoinductive bioceramics could induce tissue regeneration and, thus, is hopeful in achieving permanent restoration of damaged tissue.

In recent decades, much research has been conducted on the osteoinduction of Ca-P ceramics. One focus is on the important material factors which contribute to the osteoinductivity of the Ca-P biomaterials, as shown in Figure 3.1. Phase composition, referred to as chemical composition in some cases, was confirmed to affect the osteoinductivity. The most popular osteoinductive Ca-P ceramics include HA, β-TCP, and BCP (a mixture of HA phase and β-TCP phase with different ratios) [4, 28], and the reported osteoinductivity is in an order as BCP > β-TCP > HA >> α-TCP [29–31]. It seems that Ca-P ceramics with higher solubility could result in higher osteoinductivity, while the exception happens when the ceramic is too soluble to afford stable interface, such as β-TCP and α-TCP [32]. Macro- and micro-pore structures have been confirmed as necessary for Ca-P osteoinduction [33]. The porous structures accommodate the ingrowth of cells, and the interconnected porous channel functions to allow body fluid, blood vessels, and cells to develop toward the center of the scaffold, as well as the adequate exchange of oxygen and nutrition. Micro-pores (pore diameter <10 μm) on the walls of macro-pores allow the body's fluids to penetrate; they afford an inner rough surface for cell attachment, the adsorption of proteins [34], and the expression of osteogenic phenotype [4, 30, 35], as well as maintain the local concentration of dissolved Ca^{2+} and PO_4^{3-} and decrease the shear stresses exerted on the cells. Ca-P ceramics lacking a porous structure, such as Ca-P cements, do not show osteoinductivity [32]. Besides, other physiochemical characteristics of Ca-P bioceramics, such as bone-like apatite, nanoscale, and nanostructure [14, 36], the releasing of Ca^{2+} and PO_4^{3-}, the surface topography, as well as the surface mechanical properties, are found to be highly related to osteoinductivity. Optimizing these properties may endow the material with the function of inducing bone regeneration and, thus, enhance their bioactivity.

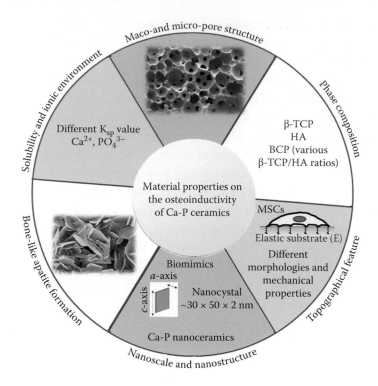

FIGURE 3.1 Material characteristics related to osteoinduction of Ca-P bioactive ceramics and hypothesis for the osteoinductive mechanism of Ca-P bioactive ceramics.

Another focus is on the mechanism of Ca-P osteoinduction. As for the biological process of bone regeneration, the microenvironment created by Ca-P bioactive ceramics benefits from the interactions between cells and matrix; subsequently, the biosignals initiate cell differentiation along the osteolineage and bone regeneration. Figure 3.2 shows the differentiation of mesenchymal stem cells (MSCs) along the osteolineage, induced by Ca-P bioactive ceramics, and the hypothesis for the osteoinductive mechanism of Ca-P, in which various interacted factors and processes have been involved. The existing theories mainly concern the adsorption of proteins and the interaction between Ca-P materials and different cells. Besides, as the osteoinduction of Ca-P involves not only the bone system but also the vascular and immune systems, a hybrid hypothesis was proposed and described as follows: first, the injury caused the invasion of the inflammatory factors and cells; second, the Ca-P ceramics work through soluble factors (such as Ca^{2+} and PO_4^{3-} ions), insoluble factors (such as their micro- or even nano-scale topographic features), and/or interact with inflammatory factors and cells, thus resulting in the adsorption and concentration of related proteins (osteogenic growth factors, cell adhesive proteins, and inflammatory factors), as well as the recruitment of various kinds of progenitor cells (monocytes, MSCs, endothelial cells, and pericytes); the process above may be accompanied with the dynamic dissolution/precipitation of Ca-P, and co-precipitation of proteins to form the bone apatite-like layer on Ca-P surface; third, there are two pathways that may lead to the osteoinduction: one is that Ca-P (as the changed form) directly stimulates the osteoblastic differentiation of MSCs;

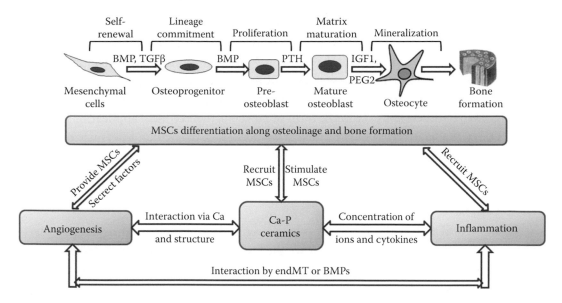

FIGURE 3.2 MSCs differentiation along osteolineage induced by Ca-P bioactive ceramics and hypothesis for the osteoinductive mechanism of Ca-P bioactive ceramics.

the other one is that Ca-P interacts with the inflammatory cells (monocytes, macrophages, and osteoclast), which result in a more osteoinductive surface and higher concentrations of Ca^{2+} and PO_4^{3-}, as well as osteogenic cytokines, and finally, these factors trigger the MSCs differentiation. The last step may involve the angiogenesis, which could interact with both the Ca-P and inflammatory response, to contribute to osteoinduction by providing more osteogenic factors and MSCs.

3.1.3 Bioactive Ceramics for Regenerative Engineering

3.1.3.1 Calcium Phosphate Bioactive Ceramics

Among various bioactive ceramics, Ca-P ceramics are undoubtedly the most promising [3, 4, 23] and have been used widely in a variety of orthopedic treatments for diseased and damaged bones. Many products have been placed on the market. One product branded as Osteoinductive Calcium Phosphate Bioceramics (BAM®) by Engineering Research Center in Biomaterials, Sichuan University, has been cleared by the State Food and Drug Administration in 2003.

The products are mainly used in non-load-bearing orthopedic repair, and the research for the optimization of bioactivity to induce full bone regeneration is still ongoing. Currently, Ca-P coating with bioactivity on biomedical metals, such as titanium (Ti) metal and its alloys, stainless steel, and Co–Cr–Mo alloys, is widely used for the load-bearing purpose and has been successfully applied in artificial hip joint and dental implants.

3.1.3.2 Bioactive Silicate Ceramics

To date, more than 20 silicate ceramics with various compositions have been prepared [37–39]. The study of bioactive silicate ceramics for bone tissue regeneration has become a hot topic. The research has focused on the ceramic preparation methods, mechanical strength, apatite mineralization, dissolution, bioactive properties and corresponding mechanism. The first and most famous silicate ceramics is Bioglass (BG), which has been approved by the Food and Drug Administration (FDA) and applied in the clinic for treating periodontal diseases and middle ear surgery. Another product branded as NovaBone® extended the application of BG to the orthopedic area [40–42]. Generally speaking, as silicate ceramics are in the form of powders, their clinical applications are still limited due to the relatively poor mechanical properties, in particular, low fracture toughness. A promising application is to deposit ceramic and glass onto the surface of Ti and its alloys to achieve excellent mechanical properties [43, 44].

3.1.3.3 Ceramic-Based Composite Scaffolds

A series of natural and synthetic polymers have been widely employed to prepare polymer–ceramic composite. The composites improve the mechanical properties more or less, while the disadvantage includes poor cell affinity and cell–matrix interaction resulting from the release of acidic degradation products.

Research also discussed adding inorganic materials in the composite scaffolds. Many types of composites such as Ca-P/Ca-Si composites and Ca-P/BG have been successfully prepared and showed higher bioactivity and more desirable degradability than those of single ceramics [45, 46].

3.1.4 Processing and Fabrication of Bioactive Ceramics for Regenerative Engineering

The bioactivity and clinical application potential of ceramics are highly dependent on the material compositions, the scaffold morphologies, and microstructure as well. The preparation of ceramics normally includes four steps, with the detailed process shown in Figure 3.3. Generally, the implants must have the shape or size matching the defects. More importantly, to endow the ceramics with bioactivity, the porous structure of the scaffold is key [6, 47–49]. Table 3.2 shows the different types of pores and their roles in biofunction restoration. Therefore, controlling pore structure is one of the most important procedures during ceramics scaffold preparation.

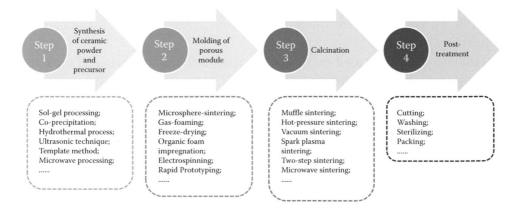

FIGURE 3.3 Normal process for the fabrication of bioactive ceramics.

TABLE 3.2   Porous Structures in Natural Cancellous Bone and Their Functions [22, 50, 51]

Pore	Size (μm)	Functions
Macro-pore	100–800	Facilitating the rapid bone ingrowth and vascularization
Minor-pore	10–100	Favorable to exchange of nutrient substances and growth of cells
Micro-pore	<10	Beneficial to the penetration of body's fluids and favorable to protein adsorption

Conventional fabrication methods of porous structure are listed in Table 3.3. Microsphere-sintering seems to be ideal because the pore size and porosity can be easily controlled, but it's difficult to produce abundant micropores, and the ceramics using this approach don't possess good bioactivity or osteoinductivity. Another feasible approach is H_2O_2 gas-foaming method, which is favorable to produce abundant micro pores besides interconnecting macro-pores. This method is low-cost, quick, and easy, but its disadvantage is that it is hard to control the porosity [3, 50].

Recently, three-dimensional (3D) printing has been employed to create complex porous ceramic matrices directly from powders [52–55], making it possible to produce bone grafts with complex shapes and internal channel networks mimicking bone structures. One of the limitations comes from the printing accuracy, including the printer controlling system and the "printing-ink." At present, it's difficult to control the microstructure on the micrometer scale. In addition, the present fabricating routines for ceramic scaffolds generally include the printing of the materials and the following sintering. Due to the shrinkage of ceramics in sintering, it's difficult to get the designed scaffolds using direct 3D printing. Future research should develop novel prototyping methods to improve the precision controlled at the micrometer, the molding method to strengthen mechanical properties, and the structural design to optimize the bioactivity of the scaffolds.

TABLE 3.3   Fabrication Methods for Three-Dimensional Porous Ceramic Scaffolds

Methods	Pore Diameter (μm)	Advantages	Disadvantages
Microsphere-sintering [56, 57]	10–1000	High mechanical properties; controlled pore size and porosity	Lack of micropores; use of template
Gas-foaming [3, 58–60]	100–800; <100	Abundant micropores; interconnecting pores, low cost	Difficultly in controlling pore structure
Freeze drying [61–63]	10–600	Biomimetic 3D porous structure	Time-consuming
Organic foam impregnation [64–67]	100–5000	Easily controlling, high porosity	Lack of micropores; low mechanical properties; use of template
Electrospinning [68–70]	0.1–50	High porosity; abundant micropores	Lack of macropores; low mechanical properties
3D printing [52–55]	50–1000	Controlled pore size and porosity; highly reproducible	Need special equipments

The sintering process is necessary for the fabrication of bioceramics with certain mechanical properties and structures. In the meantime, some microstructures could be produced by sintering such as nano-sized crystals and micro-porous structure. Traditional sintering processes include muffle sintering, hot pressure sintering, and vacuum sintering (Table 3.4). High temperature sintering would increase the mechanical strength of ceramics while, in turn, result in larger-sized crystals and denser microstructures, which are regarded as adverse to its bioactivity. Therefore, some new sintering processes such as spark plasma sintering, two-step sintering, and microwave sintering to produce ceramics with nano-crystals and increased micro pores show potential in improving the bioactivity of the ceramics.

3.2 BIOACTIVE METALS

The introduction of metal as biomaterials has been known in medical applications for a long time. In their early development, mechanical strength and corrosion were two main problems faced by metal implants. With the development of new generation biomaterials, the separate concepts of bioactive materials and biodegradable materials have converged.

With the recent development in biomaterials, a new concept of biodegradable metals (BMs) has been dramatically developed. The BMs are defined as materials used for medical implants that allow the implants to degrade in human body environment [83]. In materials science, BMs can be classified as pure metals, alloys, and metal matrix composites. Given the concerns for the biosafety of the corrosion products, the alloying elements and their quantities should be controlled without causing adverse pathophysiological and toxicological effects.

TABLE 3.4 Advantages and Disadvantages of Different Ceramic Sintering Routes

Methods	Advantages	Disadvantages
Muffle sintering [3, 71]	Inexpensive device; high yield; suitable for conventional and large size of ceramic fabrication	Time and energy consuming; unsuitable for nanoceramic fabrication
Hot pressure sintering [72, 73]	Suitable for conventional and dense ceramic fabrication; high mechanical strength	Low yield; time and energy consuming; unsuitable for nanoceramic fabrication
Vacuum sintering [74, 75]	High yield; suitable for conventional and large size of ceramic fabrication	Special equipment, time and energy consuming; unsuitable for nanoceramic fabrication
Spark plasma sintering [76–78]	Rapid process; low energy cost; suitable for nanoceramic fabrication	Expensive devices; low yield; difficult for large size of ceramic fabrication
Two-step sintering [79, 80]	Inexpensive device	Time and energy consuming; difficult for nanoceramic fabrication
Microwave sintering [3, 14, 81, 82]	Rapid process; low energy cost; suitable for nanoceramic fabrication	Expensive devices; difficult for large size of ceramic fabrication

3.2.1 Bioactive Metal with Osteoinductivity for Regenerative Engineering

From a clinical point of view, the ideal biomaterial acting as a bone substitute should possess osteoconductive and osteoinductive ability, as well as suitable mechanical properties [31, 84]. As osteoinductive biomaterials, the important factors for osteoinduction are thought to be (i) the chemical composition of the biomaterial surface and (ii) the surface morphology of the biomaterial. The formation of calcium phosphate bone-like apatite surface of the material is considered to be an important factor in osteoinductive materials. At the same time, the porous structure is considered to be an essential factor to induce bone formation. That is, all biomaterials that induce apatite layer in the body may have the potential to be osteoinductive materials when they possess a specific porous structure.

Since the 1980s, it has been reported that bioactive metals could be converted into an osteoinductive material through specific chemical and thermal treatments. It is well established that metal implants bond to living bone through an apatite layer that forms on their surfaces in the living body. The metals with bone-like apatite formation ability on its surface, when given a proper porous structure, demonstrated their osteoinductive ability [85].

Generally, Ti was reported to show that it has a superior in vitro apatite-forming ability and that it can directly bond to living bone in vivo. However, in most cases, appropriate surface treatments are necessary to modify and activate the metal surface, thus endowing a porous metal with osteoinductive bioactivity. Surface treatments may change the surface microstructure and chemical composition of porous Ti. Porous Ti with different surface treatments showed excellent ability to induce bone-like apatite formation, thus possessing in vitro bioactivity. For example, surface treatments including acid-alkali treatment, hydrogen peroxide treatment, hydrogen peroxide solution containing tantalum chloride treatment, and chemical and thermal treatments performed on porous Ti, showed varied in vitro bone-like apatite forming ability and in vivo osteoinductivity. In dorsal implantations for 3 and 5 months, ectopic bone formation was found histologically in most porous Ti metals after implantation in the thigh bone of adult dogs for 2 months (Figure 3.4). These results demonstrated that surface treatments could endow porous Ti with apatite-forming ability in vitro and induce ectopic bone formation.

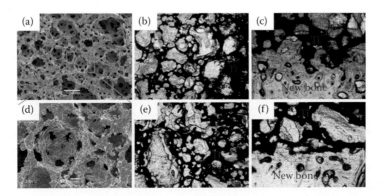

FIGURE 3.4   SEM of porous Ti metals at magnifications of (a) 35×, (d) 100×, and osteoinduction phenomenon of the porous Ti metals after implantation in the thigh bone of dogs for 2 months.

3.2.2 Biodegradable Metals for Regenerative Engineering

The concept of commercialized BM medical devices design opens an extreme new horizon and provides additional insight. Metallic biomaterials are no longer required to be inert but they should be able to assist in and promote the healing process. In practical clinical applications, several specific clinical problems (such as bone fracture and vessel blockages) need BMs for tissue healing process. The temporary support of BMs can only be provided by an implant made of degradable metals, which allow the implant to progressively degrade after fulfilling its function. Undoubtedly, with more successes emerging, BMs are becoming rising stars in the next generation of metallic biomaterials [86, 87].

3.2.2.1 Degradation Mechanism of Biodegradable Metals

As a key issue for BMs, biodegradation mechanism should be carefully investigated. In the last decade, including the corrosion mechanisms and their influencing factors, degradation rate control and ion release behavior of BMs have been widely studied [88]. The typical mode of degradation in BMs is through a corrosion process [89]. The corrosion generally proceeds by an electrochemical reaction with electrolyte to produce oxides, hydroxides, hydrogen gas, or other compounds. In the nearly neutral physiological environment, the corrosion reactions involve the following anodic dissolution of the metal and the reduction reaction (cathodic reaction); the corresponding degradation reactions are given in Equations (3.1)–(3.4):

$$\text{Oxidation reaction}: M \rightarrow M^{n+} + ne^- \tag{3.1}$$

$$\text{Reduction reaction}: 2H_2O + 2e^- \rightarrow H_2(g) + 2OH^- \tag{3.2}$$

$$\text{Reduction reaction}: 2H_2O + O_2 + 4e^- \rightarrow 4OH^- \tag{3.3}$$

$$\text{Product formation reaction}: M^{n+} + nOH^- \rightarrow M(OH)_n \tag{3.4}$$

When metals react with body fluid, they release electrons and form positive ions. In electrochemistry, the values of standard electrode potential provide a way to compare the relative ease of different metal elements to lose electrons and form ions in solutions. For biodegradable metals, they have a greater tendency to form their ions compared to hydrogen. The degradation mechanism of BMs is mainly electrochemical corrosion, and electrochemical measurements are conduced to predict the corrosion rate of BMs *in vitro*.

The biological environment has a considerable influence on the corrosion reactions of BMs. The corrosion mechanism and apatite formation process of BMs in the human biological environment are shown in Figure 3.5. From a chemical point of view, the chemical environment of blood plasma is highly soluble for BMs, especially because of the presence of a high concentration of chloride ions. Other ions present may also strongly contribute to the corrosion process. Besides, the body temperature of 37°C typically accelerates

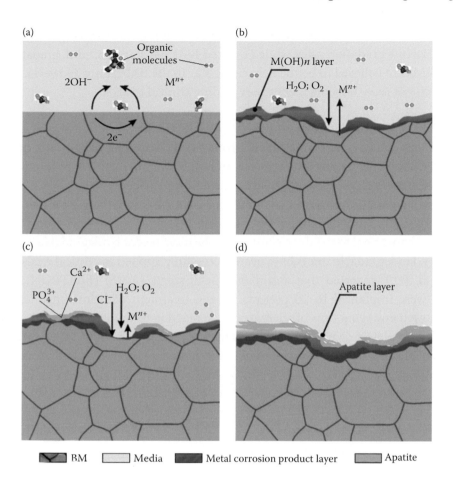

FIGURE 3.5 Corrosion mechanism and apatite formation process of BMs in human biological environment.

electrochemical reactions. Another significant factor determining the corrosion behavior of metals is the pH value. However, it is still a challenge for researchers to figure out the real corrosion mechanism of BMs in the human biological environment.

3.2.2.2 Types of Biodegradable Metals

The developed BMs include three main body systems: (i) Mg-based BMs, (ii) Fe-based BMs, and (iii) Zn-based BMs and other BMs (Ca-based and Sr-based BMGs, etc.). Table 3.5 shows some research progress for the three BM systems since 2010. It is clear that among these BMs, Mg-based BMs are the hottest topic and have been extensively published. Fe-based BMs are reported recently on alloy design and some animal testing as potential vascular stent. Zn-based BMs are studied by fewer researchers but seem to be a promising candidate in the family of BMs. Most research focuses on degradation rate controlling, in vitro cytotoxicity, and animal testing. Several Mg-based alloys have been reported and their degradation rate has been proven to be too fast and rarely homogeneous. Fe-based alloys show appropriate mechanical properties but very low degradation rate. Zn-based

BMs have corrosion rates faster than Fe, but slower than Mg. Considering Mg-based BMs need decreased degradation rates while Fe-based BMs need enhanced degradation rates, Zn-based BMs are believed to be the next rising star in the BM family. However, there has been a paucity of reports in the literature regarding clinical trials.

3.2.3 Biodegradable Metals with Clinical Application

Figure 3.6 shows two main application products of BMs, i.e., stents and orthopedic implants [113]. Stenting has become a proven procedure for the treatment of coronary artery occlusions. During this procedure, a stent is delivered and placed into a narrowed coronary artery by using a catheter system that is inserted into the artery through a small incision in the arm or groin. Since its first application in 1987 [114], stents have progressed from the conventional bare metal to the drug eluting and the most recent biodegradable stents.

Presently, biodegradable stents have been successfully applied in clinical trials. In 2005, Peeters et al. [115] reported that absorbable metal stents (AMS) (BIOTRONIK, Berlin, Germany) were implanted in 20 patients for the treatment of below-knee lesions. No patients showed any symptoms of allergic or toxic reaction to the stent material. The stents were nearly completely degraded 6 weeks after implantation. The first successful implantation of an Mg-based stent into the pulmonary artery of a preterm baby was reported by Zartner et al. in 2005 [116]. In the clinical trial, a Lekton Magic AMS by Lekton Inc. was implanted into the left pulmonary artery of a preterm baby. The degradation process

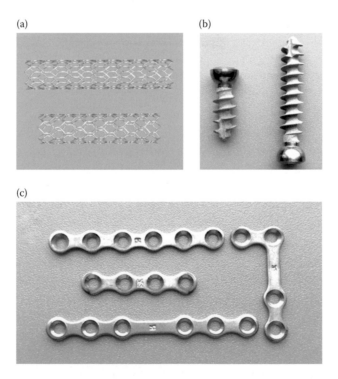

FIGURE 3.6 Two main clinical application products of BMs: (a) stents; (b) and (c) orthopedic implants.

TABLE 3.5   Some Research Progress of the Three BM Systems

Types of BMs	Materials	Published Time	Progress and Findings	Potential Applications
Mg-based BMs	ZEK100 alloys [90]	2016	Evaluate the bioabsorbable metallic biomaterial/cell interfaces that may lead to toxicity	No declaration
	Mg–Zn–Ca–Sr BMGs [91]	2016	In vitro responses of bone-forming MC3T3-E1 pre-osteoblasts to Mg–Zn–Ca–Sr BMGs were studied	No declaration
	Mg-3 wt% Zn alloy (MZ3) [92]	2016	Hot rolled Mg-3 wt% Zn alloy (MZ3) has been investigated for its potential in orthopedic implants	Orthopedic implantations
	Mg–8Er–1Zn [93]	2015	A novel Mg–8Er–1Zn alloy with the ultimate tensile strength (318 MPa), tensile yield strength (207 MPa) and elongation (21%) were reported	No declaration
	Mg60Zn35Ca5 and Mg72Zn23Ca5 [94]	2015	Used first-principles molecular dynamics simulations to elucidate the structure of Mg60Zn35Ca5 and Mg72Zn23Ca5 bulk metallic glasses	No declaration
	Nano-HA reinforced AZ31[95]	2014	Embedded nHA particles enhance the biomineralization and control the degradation	Skeletal implants
	Mg and Mg10Gd1Nd [96]	2014	Pre-incubation of material under cell culture conditions formed a natural protective layer, improved the biocompatibility of BMs	Orthopedic implantations
	AZ31/(P1, 4, 4, 4 dpp) surface coating [97]	2014	Reported a new surface coating for Mg alloy AZ31 based on a low-toxicity ionic liquid, tributyl(methyl) phosphonium diphenyl phosphate, to control its corrosion rate	Stents
	RS66 [98]	2013	In vitro and in vivo experiments were conducted to analyze the biodegradation behavior and the biocompatibility	Prosthesis implantation
	Mg–Zn [99]	2011	Conducted biocompatibility test in vitro and biodagradation in vivo	Orthopedic implantations

(*Continued*)

TABLE 3.5 *(Continued)* Some Research Progress of the Three BM Systems

Types of BMs	Materials	Published Time	Progress and Findings	Potential Applications
Fe-based BMs	Fe0.75B0.15Si0.1)100-xNbx (x=0, 1 and 3 at%) metallic glasses [100]	2016	Alloys exhibit excellent apatite-forming ability in simulated body fluids, which is expected to be applied in stents and orthopedic implants	No declaration
	Fe-based glassy alloys [101]	2016	Studied the multiple corrosion potentials alkaline solution	No declaration
	Fe-based metallic materials [102]	2015	Cytotoxicity of corrosion products of Fe-based stents relative to pH and insoluble products were studied	Stents
	Fe80-x-yCrxMoyP13C7 bulk metallic glasses [103]	2015	Alloys exhibit no cytotoxicity to NIH3T3 cells, and exhibit high corrosion resistance and excellent biocompatibility	No declaration
	Pure Fe and two alloys (Fe-10 Mn-1Pd, Fe-21 Mn-0.7C-1Pd) [104]	2014	The study investigated the degradation performance of three Fe-based materials in a growing rat skeleton over a period of 1 year	No declaration
	Fe–Mn–C–Pd alloys [105]	2013	The research studied the alloying elements' influence on metabolic processes	No declaration
	Fe–Mn–Pd alloys [106]	2010	Proposed design strategy for the development of Fe-based alloys offering both an enhanced degradation rate and suitable strength and ductility	Medical applications
	Fe(73.5)Si(13.5) B9Nb3Cu1 alloy [107]	2010	Studied the corrosion behaviors of amorphous and nanocrystalline Fe-based alloys in NaCl solution	No declaration
Zn-based BMs	Zn–Mg and two Zn–Al binary alloys [108]	2016	Alloys were developed by casting process and homogenized followed by hot extrusion. Tube extrusion was performed to produce tubes for biodegradable stents. Corrosion tests were performed using Hanks modified solution	Stents

(Continued)

TABLE 3.5 *(Continued)*   Some Research Progress of the Three BM Systems

Types of BMs	Materials	Published Time	Progress and Findings	Potential Applications
	Zn–Mg alloy [109]	2015	Zn–Mg alloys with different Mg contents were prepared by melting-casting method. The nano-structure of Zn-3 wt% Mg alloy contributes to a general corrosion	No declaration
	Zn alloys [110]	2013	Zinc exhibits ideal physiological corrosion behavior for bioabsorbable stents	Stents
	CaZn-based bulk glassy alloy [111]	2011	Develop CaZn- based glassy alloys with low Young's modulus, high fracture strength, good corrosion resistance and cytocompatibility	Orthopaedic implantations
	Zn–Mg alloys containing up to 3 wt% Mg [112]	2011	The corrosion rates of the Zn–Mg alloys were determined to be significantly lower than those of Mg and AZ91HP alloys	No declaration

had been completed 5 months after implantation. In 2007, the PROGRESS-AMS clinical trial, sponsored by BIOTRONIK GMBH& Co. (Berlin, Germany), was conducted to assess the efficacy and safety of AMSs in eight centers. A total of 71 stents, 10–15 mm in length and 3–3.5 mm in diameter, were successfully implanted after pre-dilation in 63 patients. No myocardial infarction, subacute or late thrombosis, or death occurred. In 2016, Haude et al. [117] reported the first-in-man trial (BIO-SOLVE-1), which was conducted with 46 patients at five European centers. The 12-month results showed no cardiac death or scaffold thrombosis. As the above literature had reported, the biodegradable stents had been optimized to provide better degradation resistance than their predecessors, which demonstrated full degradation in 9–12 months.

Patients with bone disease or bone fractures are commonly admitted to the clinic. Thus, fractured bone fixtures, such as plates, screws, pins, nails, wires, and needles, consisting of BMs, have become a large potential market. So far, ZEK 100, LAE 442, MgCa 0.8, and MgYREZr Mg-based alloys have been fabricated in different orthopedic applications for experimental models and clinical trials.

3.2.4 New Manufacturing and Processing Techniques of Biomedical Metals

Usually, normal manufacturing and processing methods can be applied to obtain the BMs devices. However, rather than make alloys using a traditional melting process, some nonconventional processing techniques could improve their properties.

In recent years, some advanced manufacturing technologies have been proposed in BMs fields. For instance, by using 3D printing technology, the BMs can be directly processed into scaffolds or implants. To fabricate bone scaffolds, 3D porous structures have been pursued to allow for bony ingrowth to mimic the natural porous structure of bone. It has been possible to create a controllable porous, interconnected architecture via 3D printing technology. By using 3D printing, complex, customizable parts from metal powders can be directly manufactured into scaffolds with precise porosity. Researchers believe that 3D printing will be a promising technology for manufacturing BMs products.

3.3 CONCLUDING REMARKS AND PERSPECTIVES

The development of regenerative engineering provides an effective approach for tissue repair and regeneration. The selection of scaffold material and structure optimization is important to fully mimic the 3D network structure of natural tissue. Bioactive ceramics and metals are drawing more attention due to their excellent biocompatibility and osteogenesis. Thanks to the founding of bioactive ceramics with osteoinductivity, more focus is on the design of material bioactivity to induce tissue regeneration, to realize the replacement of damaged tissue by the regenerated new tissue. To achieve the objective, on the one hand, it is necessary to explore the responding mechanism between biomaterials and cells on a molecular and genetic level to supply principles for improving material bioactivity; on the other hand, it is necessary to probe new material designs and fabrication techniques to obtain tunable and optimized mechanical and degradation properties. For metals with superior mechanical properties, a future revolution might come from biodegradable metal implants. By optimizing the bioactivity of metals to achieve specific biological function such as osteoinduction and regulation of metal degradation, biometals are also expected to be able to achieve bone tissue regeneration in the future.

REFERENCES

1. Hench, L.L. and J.M. Polak, Third-generation biomedical materials. *Science*, 2002. **295**(5557): pp.1014–1017.
2. Ma, P.X., *Biomaterials and Regenerative Medicine*. Cambridge: Cambridge University Press, 2014.
3. Hong, Y., et al., Fabrication, biological effects, and medical applications of calcium phosphate nanoceramics. *Materials Science and Engineering: R: Reports*, 2010. **70**(3): pp. 225–242.
4. Barradas, A.M., et al., Osteoinductive biomaterials: current knowledge of properties, experimental models and biological mechanisms. *European Cells & Materials*, 2011. **21**(12): pp. 4532–4545.
5. Stevens, M.M., Biomaterials for bone tissue engineering. *Materials Today*, 2008. **11**(5): pp. 18–25.
6. Schieker, M., et al., Biomaterials as scaffold for bone tissue engineering. *European Journal of Trauma*, 2006. **32**(2): pp. 114–124.
7. Ge, Z., Z. Jin, and T. Cao, Manufacture of degradable polymeric scaffolds for bone regeneration. *Biomedical Materials*, 2008. **3**(2): pp. 022001.
8. Zavan, B., et al., Hyaluronan based porous nano-particles enriched with growth factors for the treatment of ulcers: a placebo-controlled study. *Journal of Materials Science: Materials in Medicine*, 2009. **20**(1): pp. 235–247.
9. Vasanthan, K.S., et al., Role of biomaterials, therapeutic molecules and cells for hepatic tissue engineering. *Biotechnology Advances*, 2012. **30**(3): pp. 742–752.

10. Shuai, C., et al., Structure and properties of nano-hydroxypatite scaffolds for bone tissue engineering with a selective laser sintering system. *Nanotechnology*, 2011. **22**(28): pp. 285703.

11. Chai, Y.C., et al., Current views on calcium phosphate osteogenicity and the translation into effective bone regeneration strategies. *Acta Biomaterialia*, 2012. **8**(11): pp. 3876–3887.

12. Akao, M., H. Aoki, and K. Kato, Mechanical properties of sintered hydroxyapatite for prosthetic applications. *Journal of Materials Science*, 1981. **16**(3): pp. 809–812.

13. Orlovskii, V., V. Komlev, and S. Barinov, Hydroxyapatite and hydroxyapatite-based ceramics. *Inorganic Materials*, 2002. **38**(10): pp. 973–984.

14. Li, B., et al., Fabrication and cellular biocompatibility of porous carbonated biphasic calcium phosphate ceramics with a nanostructure. *Acta Biomaterialia*, 2009. **5**(1): pp. 134–143.

15. Thompson, I. and L. Hench, Mechanical properties of bioactive glasses, glass-ceramics and composites. *Proceedings of the Institution of Mechanical Engineers, Part H: Journal of Engineering in Medicine*, 1998. **212**(2): pp. 127–136.

16. Vitalebrovarone, C., F. Baino, and E. Verné, High strength bioactive glass-ceramic scaffolds for bone regeneration. *Journal of Materials Science Materials in Medicine*, 2009. **20**(2): pp. 643–653.

17. Wu, C. and J. Chang, A review of bioactive silicate ceramics. *Biomedical Materials*, 2013. **8**(3): pp. 032001.

18. Kikuchi, M., et al., Self-organization mechanism in a bone-like hydroxyapatite/collagen nanocomposite synthesized in vitro and its biological reaction in vivo. *Biomaterials*, 2001. **22**(13): pp. 1705–1711.

19. Losquadro, W., S. Tatum, M.J. Allen, and K. Mann, Polylactide-co-glycolide fiber-reinforced calcium phosphate bone cement. *Archives of Facial Plastic Surgery*, 2009. **11**(2): pp. 104–109.

20. Salinas, A. and M. Valletregi, Bioactive ceramics: from bone grafts to tissue engineering. *RSC Advances*, 2013. **3**(28): pp. 11116–11131.

21. Liu, X., et al., Bioactive calcium silicate ceramics and coatings. *Biomedecine Pharmacotherapy*, 2008. **62**(8): pp. 526–529.

22. Wang, J., et al., Effect of phase composition on protein adsorption and osteoinduction of porous calcium phosphate ceramics in mice. *Journal of Biomedical Materials Research Part A*, 2014. **102**(12): pp. 4234–4243.

23. Li, X., et al., Influences of the steam sterilization on the properties of calcium phosphate porous bioceramics. *Journal of Materials Science Materials in Medicine*, 2016. **27**(1): pp. 1–10.

24. Cao, H. and N. Kuboyama, A biodegradable porous composite scaffold of PGA/β-TCP for bone tissue engineering. *Bone*, 2009. **46**(2): pp. 386–395.

25. Hou, Z., et al., Preparation and properties of poly(L-lactide-co-glycolide). *Journal of Biomedical Engineering Research*, 2014. **33**(1): pp. 29–31.

26. Yuan, H., et al., Osteoinductive ceramics as synthetic alternative to autologous bone grafting. *Proceedings of the National Academy of Sciences of the United States of America*, 2010. **107**(31): pp. 13614–13619.

27. Urist, M.R., A. Mikulski, and A. Lietze, Solubilized and insolubilized bone morphogenetic protein. *Proceedings of the National Academy of Sciences*, 1979. **76**(4): pp. 1828–1832.

28. Wang, Z., et al., Applications of calcium phosphate nanoparticles in porous hard tissue engineering scaffolds. *Nano*, 2012. **7**(4): pp. 12304-1–12304-18.

29. Yuan, H., et al., Bone formation induced by calcium phosphate ceramics in soft tissue of dogs: a comparative study between porous α-TCP and β-TCP. *Journal of Materials Science Materials in Medicine*, 2001. **12**(1): pp. 7–13.

30. Samavedi, S., A.R. Whittington, and A.S. Goldstein, Calcium phosphate ceramics in bone tissue engineering: a review of properties and their influence on cell behavior. *Acta Biomaterialia*, 2013. **9**(9): pp. 8037–8045.

31. Yuan, H., et al., A comparison of the osteoinductive potential of two calcium phosphate ceramics implanted intramuscularly in goats. *Journal of Materials Science: Materials in Medicine*, 2002. **13**(12): pp. 1271–1275.

32. Yuan, H., et al., Tissue responses of calcium phosphate cement: a study in dogs. *Biomaterials*, 2000. **21**(12): pp. 1283–1290.

33. Yuan, H., et al., Osteoinduction by calcium phosphate biomaterials. *Journal of Materials Science: Materials in Medicine*, 1998. **9**(12): pp. 723–726.

34. Zhu, X.D. and H.Y. Fan, Effect of surface structure on protein adsorption to biphasic calcium-phosphate ceramics in vitro and in vivo. *Acta Biomaterialia*, 2009. **5**(4): pp. 1311–1318.

35. Zhang, X., et al., A calcium phosphate, bioceramics with osteoinduction. In *The 4th World Biomaterials Congress*, Berlin, Germany. 1992.

36. Xu, A.W., Y. Ma, and H. Cölfen, Biomimetic mineralization. *Journal of Materials Chemistry*, 2007. **17**(5): pp. 415–449.

37. Hsi, C.S., et al., Crystallization kinetics and magnetic properties of iron oxide contained $25Li_2O–8MnO_2–20CaO–2P_2O_5–45SiO_2$ glasses. *Journal of the European Ceramic Society*, 2007. **27**(10): pp. 3171–3176.

38. O'Donnell, M.D. and R.G. Hill, Influence of strontium and the importance of glass chemistry and structure when designing bioactive glasses for bone regeneration. *Acta Biomaterialia*, 2010. **6**(7): pp. 2382–2385.

39. Padilla, S., et al., Hydroxyapatite/SiO_2–CaO–P_2O_5 glass materials: in vitro bioactivity and biocompatibility. *Acta Biomaterialia*, 2006. **2**(3): pp. 331–342.

40. Juhasz, J.A. and S.M. Best, Bioactive ceramics: processing, structures and properties. *Journal of Materials Science*, 2012. **47**(2): pp. 610–624.

41. Jones, J.R., ch. 3 – Bioactive ceramics and glasses. *Tissue Engineering Using Ceramics & Polymers*, 2007. **1**: pp. 52–71.

42. Pantano Jr., C.G., A.E. Clark Jr., and L.L. Hench, Multilayer corrosion films on bioglass surfaces. *Journal of the American Ceramic Society*, 1974. **57**(9): pp. 412–413.

43. Hench, L.L., A.E. Clark, and H.F. Schaake, Effects of microstructure on the radiation stability of amorphous semiconductors ☆. *Journal of Non-Crystalline Solids*, 1972. **8**(4): pp. 837–843.

44. Piotrowski, G., et al., Mechanical studies of the bone bioglass interfacial bond. *Journal of Biomedical Materials Research*, 1975. **9**(4): pp. 47–61.

45. Hesaraki, S., M. Safari, and M.A. Shokrgozar, Development of β-tricalcium phosphate/sol-gel derived bioactive glass composites: physical, mechanical, and in vitro biological evaluations. *Journal of Biomedical Materials Research Part B: Applied Biomaterials*, 2009. **91**(1): pp. 459–469.

46. Lin, K., et al., Fabrication and characterization of hydroxyapatite/wollastonite composite bioceramics with controllable properties for hard tissue repair. *Journal of the American Ceramic Society*, 2011. **94**(1): pp. 99–105.

47. Chen, Y., et al., Enhanced effect of β-tricalcium phosphate phase on neovascularization of porous calcium phosphate ceramics: in vitro and in vivo evidence. *Acta Biomaterialia*, 2015. **11**: pp. 435–448.

48. Price, C.H.G., Book review bones and joints (monographs in pathology—No. 17). Edited by Ackerman L.V., Spjut H.J., and Abell M.R., pp. xi+349, 190 illus., 1976 (Baltimore, The Williams and Wilkins Company), £27·00. *British Journal of Radiology*, 1977. **50**(593): p. 311.

49. And, S.W. and H.D. Wagner, The material bone: structure mechanical function relations. *Annual Review of Materials Research*, 2003. **28**(1): pp. 271–298.

50. Li, X., et al., Gelatinizing technology combined with gas foaming to fabricate porous spherical hydroxyapatite bioceramic granules. *Materials Letters*, 2016. **185**: pp. 428–431.

51. Chen, H., et al., Fabrication of porous titanium scaffolds by stack sintering of microporous titanium spheres produced with centrifugal granulation technology. *Materials Science & Engineering C*, 2014. **43**: pp. 182–188.

52. Inzana, J.A., et al., 3D printing of composite calcium phosphate and collagen scaffolds for bone regeneration. *Biomaterials*, 2014. **35**(13): pp. 4026–4034.

53. Trombetta, R., et al., 3D printing of calcium phosphate ceramics for bone tissue engineering and drug delivery. *Annals of Biomedical Engineering*, 2016. 45(1): pp. 1–22.

54. Khalyfa, A., et al., Development of a new calcium phosphate powder-binder system for the 3D printing of patient specific implants. *Journal of Materials Science: Materials in Medicine*, 2007. **18**(5): pp. 909–916.

55. Bergmann, C., et al., 3D printing of bone substitute implants using calcium phosphate and bioactive glasses. *Journal of the European Ceramic Society*, 2010. **30**(12): pp. 2563–2567.

56. Descamps, M., et al., Synthesis of macroporous β-tricalcium phosphate with controlled porous architectural. *Ceramics International*, 2008. **34**(5): pp. 1131–1137.

57. Descamps, M., et al., Manufacture of macroporous β-tricalcium phosphate bioceramics. *Journal of the European Ceramic Society*, 2008. **28**(1): pp. 149–157.

58. Ryshkewitch, E., Compression strength of porous sintered alumina and zirconia. *Journal of the American Ceramic Society*, 2006. **36**(2): pp. 65–68.

59. Engin, N.O. and A.C. Tas, Manufacture of macroporous calcium hydroxyapatite bioceramics. *Journal of the European Ceramic Society*, 1999. **19**(13–14): pp. 2569–2572.

60. Aritaa, I.H., et al., Chemistry and sintering behaviour of thin hydroxyapatite ceramics with controlled porosity. *Biomaterials*, 1995. **16**(5): pp. 403–408.

61. Fu, Q., et al., Freeze-spray deposition of layered alumina/zirconia composites. *Materials Science & Engineering B*, 2009. **161**(1–3): pp. 120–124.

62. Fu, Q., et al., Freeze casting of porous hydroxyapatite scaffolds. I. Processing and general microstructure. *Journal of Biomedical Materials Research Part B: Applied Biomaterials*, 2008. **86**(1): pp. 125–135.

63. Deville, S., E. Saiz, and A.P. Tomsia, Freeze casting of hydroxyapatite scaffolds for bone tissue engineering. *Biomaterials*, 2006. **27**(32): pp. 5480–5489.

64. Liu, B., et al., Porous bioceramics reinforced by coating gelatin. *Journal of Materials Science Materials in Medicine*, 2008. **19**(3): pp. 1203–1207.

65. Yang, X. and Z. Wang, Synthesis of biphasic ceramics of hydroxyapatite and β-tricalcium phosphate with controlled phase content and porosity. *Journal of Materials Chemistry*, 1998. **8**(10): pp. 2233–2237.

66. Tian, J. and J. Tian, Preparation of porous hydroxyapatite. *Journal of Materials Science*, 2001. **36**(12): pp. 3061–3066.

67. Peng, H.X., et al., Microstructure of ceramic foams. *Journal of the European Ceramic Society*, 2000. **20**(7): pp. 807–813.

68. Erisken, C., D.M. Kalyon, and H. Wang, Functionally graded electrospun polycaprolactone and β-tricalcium phosphate nanocomposites for tissue engineering applications. *Biomaterials*, 2008. **29**(30): pp. 4065–4073.

69. Hong, Y., et al., Synthesis using electrospinning and stabilization of single layer macroporous films and fibrous networks of poly(vinyl alcohol). *Journal of Membrane Science*, 2006. **276**(1–2): pp. 1–7.

70. Hong, Y., H. Fan, and X. Zhang, Synthesis and protein adsorption of hierarchical nanoporous ultrathin fibers. *Journal of Physical Chemistry B*, 2009. **113**(17): pp. 5837–5842.

71. Champion, E., Sintering of calcium phosphate bioceramics. *Acta Biomaterialia*, 2013. **9**(4): pp. 5855–5875.

72. Li, P., I.-W. Chen, and J.E. Penner-Hahn, X-ray-absorption studies of zirconia polymorphs. I. Characteristic local structures. *Physical Review B*, 1993. **48**(14): pp. 10063.

73. Veljović, D., et al., Processing of dense nanostructured HAP ceramics by sintering and hot pressing. *Ceramics International*, 2009. **35**(4): pp. 1407–1413.

74. Ducheyne, P., et al., Calcium phosphate ceramic coatings on porous titanium: effect of structure and composition on electrophoretic deposition, vacuum sintering and in vitro dissolution. *Biomaterials*, 1990. **11**(4): pp. 244–254.

75. Wang, P.E. and T. Chaki, Sintering behaviour and mechanical properties of hydroxyapatite and dicalcium phosphate. *Journal of Materials Science: Materials in Medicine*, 1993. **4**(2): pp. 150–158.

76. Gu, Y., et al., Spark plasma sintering of hydroxyapatite powders. *Biomaterials*, 2002. **23**(1): pp. 37–43.
77. Xu, J., et al., Radio frequency (rf) plasma spheroidized HA powders: powder characterization and spark plasma sintering behavior. *Biomaterials*, 2005. **26**(15): pp. 2197–2207.
78. Li, W. and L. Gao, Fabrication of HAp–ZrO2 (3Y) nano-composite by SPS. *Biomaterials*, 2003. **24**(6): pp. 937–940.
79. Chen, I.-W. and X.-H. Wang, Sintering dense nanocrystalline ceramics without final-stage grain growth. *Nature*, 2000. **404**(6774): pp. 168–171.
80. Lin, K., L. Chen, and J. Chang, Fabrication of dense hydroxyapatite nanobioceramics with enhanced mechanical properties via two-step sintering process. *International Journal of Applied Ceramic Technology*, 2012. **9**(3): pp. 479–485.
81. Wang, X., et al., Fabrication and characterization of porous hydroxyapatite/β-tricalcium phosphate ceramics by microwave sintering. *Materials Letters*, 2006. **60**(4): pp. 455–458.
82. Rameshbabu, N. and K.P. Rao, Microwave synthesis, characterization and in-vitro evaluation of nanostructured biphasic calcium phosphates. *Current Applied Physics*, 2009. **9**(1): pp. S29–S31.
83. Hermawan, H., D. Dube, and D. Mantovani, Developments in metallic biodegradable stents. *Acta Biomaterialia*, 2010. **6**(5): pp. 1693–1697.
84. Jang, J.W., et al., Osteoinductive activity of biphasic calcium phosphate with different rhBMP-2 doses in rats. *Oral Surgery, Oral Medicine, Oral Pathology, and Oral Radiology*, 2012. **113**(4): pp. 480–487.
85. Kokubo, T. and S. Yamaguchi, Growth of novel ceramic layers on metals via chemical and heat treatments for inducing various biological functions. *Frontiers in Bioengineering and Biotechnology*, 2015. **3**: pp. 176.
86. Kusnierczyk, K. and M. Basista, Recent advances in research on magnesium alloys and magnesium-calcium phosphate composites as biodegradable implant materials. *Journal of Biomaterials Applications*, 2016. 31(6): pp. 878–900.
87. Seitz, J.M., et al., Recent advances in biodegradable metals for medical sutures: a critical review. *Advanced Healthcare Materials*, 2015. **4**(13): pp. 1915–1936.
88. Bajger, P., et al., Mathematical modelling of the degradation behaviour of biodegradable metals. *Biomechanics and Modeling in Mechanobiology*, 2017. **16**(1): pp. 227–238.
89. Zheng, Y.F., X.N. Gu, and F. Witte, Biodegradable metals. *Materials Science and Engineering R*, 2014. **77**: pp. 1–34.
90. Grillo, C.A., F. Alvarez, and M.A. Fernandez Lorenzo de Mele, Degradation of bioabsorbable Mg-based alloys: assessment of the effects of insoluble corrosion products and joint effects of alloying components on mammalian cells. *Materials Science and Engineering C: Materials for Biological Applications*, 2016. **58**: pp. 372–380.
91. Li, H., et al., In vitro responses of bone-forming MC3T3-E1 pre-osteoblasts to biodegradable Mg-based bulk metallic glasses. *Materials Science and Engineering C: Materials for Biological Applications*, 2016. **68**: pp. 632–641.
92. Nayak, S., et al., Strengthening of Mg based alloy through grain refinement for orthopaedic application. *Journal of the Mechanical Behavior of Biomedical Materials*, 2016. **59**: pp. 57–70.
93. Zhang, J., et al., New horizon for high performance Mg-based biomaterial with uniform degradation behavior: Formation of stacking faults. *Scientific Reports*, 2015. **5**: pp. 13933.
94. Christie, J.K., Atomic structure of biodegradable Mg-based bulk metallic glass. *Physical Chemistry Chemical Physics*, 2015. **17**(19): pp. 12894–12898.
95. Ratna Sunil, B., et al., Nano-hydroxyapatite reinforced AZ31 magnesium alloy by friction stir processing: a solid state processing for biodegradable metal matrix composites. *Journal of Materials Science: Materials in Medicine*, 2014. **25**(4): pp. 975–988.
96. Willumeit, R., A. Möhring, and F. Feyerabend, Optimization of cell adhesion on mg based implant materials by pre-incubation under cell culture conditions. *International Journal of Molecular Sciences*, 2014. **15**: pp. 7639–7650.

97. Zhang, Y., M. Forsyth, and B.R. Hinton, The effect of treatment temperature on corrosion resistance and hydrophilicity of an ionic liquid coating for Mg-based stents. *ACS Applied Materials & Interfaces*, 2014. **6**(21): pp. 18989–18997.

98. Willbold, E., et al., Biocompatibility of rapidly solidified magnesium alloy RS66 as a temporary biodegradable metal. *Acta Biomaterialia*, 2013. **9**(10): pp. 8509–8517.

99. Chen, D., et al., Biocompatibility of magnesium-zinc alloy in biodegradable orthopedic implants. *International Journal of Molecular Medicine*, 2011. **28**(3): pp. 343–348.

100. Qin, C., et al., Novel bioactive Fe-based metallic glasses with excellent apatite-forming ability. *Materials Science and Engineering C: Materials for Biological Applications*, 2016. **69**: pp. 513–521.

101. Li, Y.J., et al., A practical anodic and cathodic curve intersection model to understand multiple corrosion potentials of Fe-based glassy alloys in OH-contained solutions. *PLoS One*, 2016. **11**(1): pp. e0146421.

102. Fagali, N.S., et al., Cytotoxicity of corrosion products of degradable Fe-based stents: relevance of pH and insoluble products. *Colloids and Surface B: Biointerfaces*, 2015. **128**: pp. 480–488.

103. Li, S., et al., Development of Fe-based bulk metallic glasses as potential biomaterials. *Materials Science and Engineering C: Materials for Biological Applications*, 2015. **52**: pp. 235–241.

104. Kraus, T., et al., Biodegradable Fe-based alloys for use in osteosynthesis: outcome of an in vivo study after 52 weeks. *Acta Biomaterialia*, 2014. **10**(7): pp. 3346–3353.

105. Schinhammer, M., et al., On the cytocompatibility of biodegradable Fe-based alloys. *Materials Science and Engineering C: Materials for Biological Applications*, 2013. **33**(2): pp. 782–789.

106. Schinhammer, M., et al., Design strategy for biodegradable Fe-based alloys for medical applications. *Acta Biomaterialia*, 2010. **6**(5): pp. 1705–1713.

107. Li, X., et al., Corrosion behaviors of amorphous and nanocrystalline Fe-based alloys in NaCl solution. *Journal of Nanoscience and Nanotechnology*, 2010. **10**(11): pp. 7226–7230.

108. Mostaed, E., et al., Novel Zn-based alloys for biodegradable stent applications: design, development and in vitro degradation. *Journal of the Mechanical Behavior of Biomedical Materials*, 2016. **60**: pp. 581–602.

109. Gao, W., et al., Effects of Mg on microstructure and corrosion properties of Zn–Mg alloy. *Journal of Alloys & Compounds*, 2014. **602**(5): pp. 101–107.

110. Bowen, P.K., J. Drelich, and J. Goldman, Zinc exhibits ideal physiological corrosion behavior for bioabsorbable stents. *Advance Materials*, 2013. **25**(18): pp. 2577–2582.

111. Jiao, W., et al., Development of CaZn based glassy alloys as potential biodegradable bone graft substitute. *Journal of Non-Crystalline Solids*, 2011. **357**: pp. 3830–3840.

112. Vojtech, D., et al., Mechanical and corrosion properties of newly developed biodegradable Zn-based alloys for bone fixation. *Acta Biomaterialia*, 2011. **7**(9): pp. 3515–3522.

113. Ding, W., Opportunities and challenges for the biodegradable magnesium alloys as next-generation biomaterials. *Regenerative Biomaterials*, 2016. **3**: pp. 79–86.

114. Sigwart, U., et al., Intravascular stents to prevent occlusion and restenosis after transluminal angioplasty. *New England Journal of Medicine*, 1987. **316**(12): pp. 701–706.

115. Peeters, P., et al., Preliminary results after application of absorbable metal stents in patients with critical limb ischemia. *Journal of Endovascular Therapy*, 2005. **12**(1): pp. 1–5.

116. Zartner, P., et al., First successful implantation of a biodegradable metal stent into the left pulmonary artery of a preterm baby. *Catheterization and Cardiovascular Interventions*, 2005. **66**(4): pp. 590–594.

117. Haude, M., et al., Safety and performance of the DRug-Eluting Absorbable Metal Scaffold (DREAMS) in patients with de novo coronary lesions: 3-year results of the prospective, multicentre, first-in-man BIOSOLVE-I trial. *EuroIntervention*, 2016. **12**(2): pp. e160–e166.

CHAPTER 4

Substrate Guided Cell Behavior in Regenerative Engineering

Mengqian Liu and Shyni Varghese

University of California

CONTENTS

4.1 INTRODUCTION

Stem cells hold enormous potential for a broad spectrum of applications in regenerative engineering – from *in vitro* technological platforms and model systems to cell-based therapies – owing to their ability to self-renew and differentiate into a wide range of specialized cell types. The interaction of stem cells with their surrounding microenvironment is fundamental to multiple cellular processes such as cell migration, proliferation, differentiation, and tissue homeostasis.[1–4] Historically, considerable emphasis has been placed on using soluble regulators to control stem cell fate and commitment, but studies over the last two decades have shown that the "insoluble" component, the extracellular matrix (ECM), plays an equally important role in regulating various cellular functions, including stem cell growth and differentiation. The ECM has been recognized as a reservoir of biochemical and biophysical signals that actively mediates various cellular processes, contributing to tissue morphogenesis, homeostasis, and regeneration.[5] When the ECM is perturbed, those same interactions could contribute to many diseases like cancer[6–8] and fibrosis.[9]

Biomaterials have been widely used as artificial ECM to study stem cell behaviors.[10,11] Recent research has established that material-specific properties, including biochemical signals (e.g., immobilized growth factors or functional groups),[12–16] mechanical stimuli (e.g., elastic modulus and viscoelastic properties),[17–20] and topographical signals (e.g., pores, geometry, and fibrils),[21–24] have a profound impact on stem cell growth and differentiation. In short, stem cells in contact with biomaterials can sense their surrounding and initiate elaborate intracellular signaling, which eventually translates into coherent information that regulates downstream gene and protein expression. Successful manipulation of these biomaterial-based cues has been used as a promising approach to control stem cell differentiation and facilitate the application of stem cells in regenerative engineering and generation of functional three-dimensional (3D) tissues.

In this chapter, we discuss current research findings in the design of extracellular matrix analogues to guide stem cell responses, and review the subsets of tunable materials properties that are shown to affect cellular phenotype and functions.

4.2 DESIGNING BIOMATERIALS TO CONTROL CELL FUNCTIONS

Both natural and synthetic biomaterials have been extensively studied as artificial ECMs to guide adhesion, shape, proliferation, and differentiation of stem cells. In general, native ECM-derived materials like collagen, fibronectin, and gelatin are obvious choices because of their intrinsic ability to interact with cells through features such as the presence of cell surface receptor-binding ligands, growth factors, fibrils (in the case of collagen), and susceptibility to proteolytic degradation. Despite these advantages, natural materials often suffer from issues including weak mechanical properties, high cost, potential immunogenicity, short shelf life, and batch-to-batch variability.[10] In contrast, synthetic biomaterials can be easily processed, and their physical and biochemical properties can be tailored to achieve the desired features in a spatiotemporal manner.[25,26] Synthetic materials also elicit minimal immunogenicity. Hence, hybrid materials possessing the biochemical functions of native materials and tunable physical properties of synthetic materials could be ideal candidates for cell culture.

4.2.1 Functionalizing Synthetic Materials with Cell-Adhesive Moieties

Given the propensity of ECM proteins to promote cell-matrix interactions, the functionalization of synthetic biomaterials with proteins or peptides, through either physical blending or chemical conjugation, has been widely used to promote attachment, proliferation, and even differentiation of stem cells.[12–15,27,28] For instance, synthetic matrices modified with several ECM-derived proteins such as laminin (and their isoforms) and vitronectin have been shown to support human pluripotent stem cell expansion *in vitro*.[27,28] Although ECM proteins are ideal for improving cell-matrix interactions, they can be easily denatured when exposed to the nonphysiological environment. To circumvent these limitations, peptides instead of proteins can be used to achieve similar functions.[29] Many studies have reported the use of peptide-modified biomaterials to support stem cell phenotypes.[30–32] For instance, Melkoumian *et al.* reported synthetic peptide-acrylate surfaces (PAS) as supporting self-renewal of human embryonic stem cells (hESCs) without karyotypic instability in a chemically defined, xeno-free medium condition.[31] In a similar approach, Klim *et al.* identified that a vitronectin-derived peptide sequence, GKKQRFRHRNRKG, could sustain pluripotency and self-renewal of hESCs, where the peptide sequence is shown to engage with the cells through cell surface glycans.[30] Similar strategies have also been applied to guide stem cell differentiation. Incorporation of peptide sequence KLER (lysine-leucine-glutamic acid-arginine), a collagen II binding domain derived from decorin, was shown to promote chondrogenic differentiation of human mesenchymal stem cells (hMSCs) in polyethylene glycol (PEG) hydrogels.[33] Specifically, incorporation of KLER was found to inhibit collagenase-mediated degradation of cartilage matrices and regulate transforming growth factor- β (TGF-β) signaling by stabilizing the triple-helical structure of collagen type II. The biological activity of immobilized peptides depends on their accessibility, suggesting that optimal orientation and distribution of the tethered ligands are necessary to achieve the desired functions.[34–37] Hyaluronic acid (HA), an ECM polysaccharide known to interact with cell surface receptors such as CD44, has also been extensively studied for cartilage tissue engineering from stem cells.[38–40]

4.2.2 Biomaterials to Regulate Growth Factor Signaling

Native ECM serves as a reservoir for various growth factors. The extent of growth factor sequestration varies and could have a significant influence on maintaining tissue-specific growth factor signaling. The establishment of a well-controlled growth factor milieu within a synthetic environment is crucial for controlling various cellular functions, including pluripotency and differentiation.[21]

Studies have used the inherent ability of ECM glycosaminoglycans (GAGs) to sequester growth factors through noncovalent interactions. In this regard, biomaterials were either functionalized with GAG molecules[41] or GAG mimetics.[42–43] GAG moieties strongly and reversibly bind to various morphogens, including fibroblast growth factors (FGFs), vascular endothelial growth factor (VEGF), wingless-type MMTV integration site family, member 3a, TGF-βs and insulin-like growth factors.[44–48] Moreover, the binding of proteins to GAGs increases growth factors' half-lives both *in vitro* and *in vivo* by protecting them from enzymatic degradation and environmental denaturation agents.[49–51] Several studies have used the immobilization of heparin molecules, such as PEG-heparin hydrogels, to promote differentiation of stem cells.[46] Biomaterials that sequester growth factors have also been shown to promote *in vivo* survival and engraftment of transplanted cells.[52,53] Kabra *et al.* reported that the use of HA molecules grafted with 6-aminocaproic acid (6ACA) moieties (HA-6ACA) not only improves the survival of the transplanted hESC-derived cells in skeletal muscle but also promotes their differentiation into tissue-specific cells *in vivo*.[52] It was hypothesized that the HA-6ACA molecules effectively sequester endogenous basic fibroblast growth factors (bFGFs), a key biomolecule involved in postnatal myogenesis and skeletal muscle homeostasis, and regulate their *in vivo* signaling. Immobilization of 6ACA molecules facilitates sequestration of growth factor via electrostatic interactions between the terminal carboxyl group of the 6ACA and the positively charged amino acid domain on the bFGF surface.

Studies have used synthetic heparin mimetic molecules such as polysodium-4-styrenesulfonate (PSS) to regulate the activities of growth factors such as bFGF.[42–43] Chang *et al.* have modified polyacrylamide (PAm) substrates via covalent cross-linking with PSS, and demonstrated the ability of the PAm-PSS hydrogels to support long-term expansion (≥20 passages) of hESCs and human induced pluripotent stem cells (hiPSCs), in part, owing to the potential sequestration of FGF-2 by the matrices.[42] Similarly, Hudalla *et al.* recently described covalent tethering of heparin binding peptide HEPpep, derived from the heparin binding domain of FGF-2, to oligoethylene glycol self-assembling monolayers.[54] These peptide-modified structures have been shown to sequester serum-borne heparin to modulate the presentation and availability of morphogens in the culture, resulting in increased human umbilical vein endothelial cells and mesenchymal stem cell (MSC) proliferation.

4.2.3 Biomaterial Chemistry-Mediated Cellular Responses

Besides incorporating molecular recognition elements such as peptides, proteins, or growth factors into biomaterials, studies have also used chemical functional groups to regulate various cellular behaviors. In the absence of active adhesive moieties, interfacial or chemical properties of biomaterials play a crucial role in cell-matrix interaction by mediating nonspecific adsorption of proteins. Both the functional groups and hydrophobicity of the interface have been shown to play key roles in the distribution and binding of proteins, and consequently, the attachment, growth, and differentiation of stem cells.[13,22]

Early evidence has shown that simple functional groups (e.g., OH, CH_3, NH_2, SH, and COOH) tethered on substrate surfaces appear sufficient to elicit preferential differentiation of stem cells. Curran *et al.* showed that chondrogenesis of hMSC was enhanced on OH and COOH-modified glass surfaces, whereas NH_2 and SH-modified surfaces were found to upregulate osteogenesis, and untreated and CH_3-modified surfaces supported the maintenance of undifferentiated states of MSCs.[55] In a similar study, enhanced osteogenic differentiation of MC3T3-E1 cells was observed on self-assembled monolayer surfaces modified with OH and NH_2 functional groups, compared to those functionalized with COOH and CH_3 groups.[56] The authors demonstrated a functional group's dependent activity of cell surface integrins. Specifically, selective engagement of cell surface $\alpha_5\beta_1$ integrins was present on surfaces displaying OH and NH_2 groups, an engagement of both $\alpha_5\beta_1$ and $\alpha_V\beta_3$ integrins on surfaces with COOH groups, whereas minimal engagement of either integrin on CH_3 surface was observed. Notably, the latter is due to the surface chemistry-mediated exposure of integrin binding sites of the fibronectin at the biomaterial surface.[56] These surface chemistry-dependent differences in integrin activation differentially regulated focal adhesion and subsequent intracellular signaling.[57] Interestingly, mineralization (and, hence, osteogenesis) was observed only on NH_2 and OH-modified surfaces. The β_1-blocking antibody greatly inhibited mineralization on both OH and NH_2 surfaces, while treatment with β_3-blocking antibody on COOH and NH_2 surfaces instead promoted mineralization. These findings suggest that binding of integrin $\alpha_5\beta_1$ upregulates osteogenic differentiation of the cells while $\alpha_V\beta_3$ downregulates it.[56]

In another study, Benoit *et al.* have utilized chemical functional groups of the hydrogel matrices to promote differentiation of encapsulated MSCs in a 3D culture.[58] Incorporation of small chemical groups (carboxyl, phosphate, and t-butyl groups) into PEG hydrogels preferentially drove encapsulated MSCs to differentiate via osteogenic, adipogenic, or chondrogenic pathways. Specifically, MSCs in PEG hydrogel with phosphate groups showed increased expressions of *RUNX2* and *CBFA1*, produced a collagen-rich pericellular matrix, and synthesized more osteopontin, while those exposed to *t*-butyl groups became adipogenic instead, manifested by upregulation of peroxisome proliferator-activated receptor-gamma (PPARγ) (an adipogenic marker) and intracellular lipid deposition (Figure 4.1).[58]

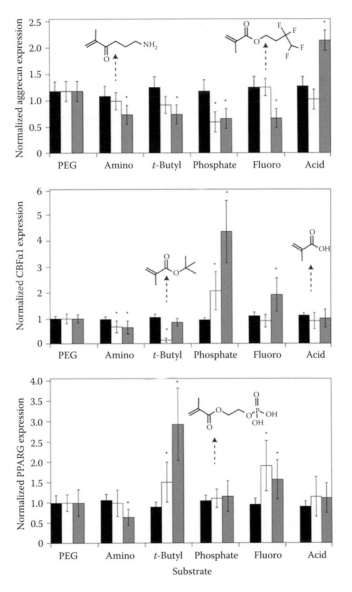

FIGURE 4.1 Gene expression profiles of aggrecan, CBFα1, and PPARγ for hMSCs seeded on surfaces modified with various functional groups, normalized to expression on control surface of unmodified PEG on days 0 (black bars), 4 (white bars), and 10 (gray bars) of culture.[58] Adapted from Mann (58), with permission, Copyright Nature Publishing Group, 2008.

4.2.4 Mineralization of Biomaterials for Bone-Specific Biochemical Cues

Biomineralization refers to modifications of organic matrices by incorporation of crystalline/semicrystalline inorganic minerals, such as calcium phosphate (CaP), to emulate the mineralization processes that occur in nature.[59-61] A popular method to achieve this is by introducing polymeric substrates with anionic polar groups to mineral ion-rich environments, such as simulated body fluid.[61-63] Upon exposure to such environments, the functional groups of the biomaterials bind calcium ions to mediate apatite nucleation and growth. Such formed mineralized biomaterials tend to exhibit better integration between the inorganic and organic components compared to organic matrices that are physically loaded CaP minerals within. In addition to functional groups, other physical parameters such as hydrophobicity of the biomaterials also play an important role in binding functional groups to inorganic ions.[61,64,65]

Several studies have indicated that biomaterials containing CaP moieties are able to promote *in vitro* osteogenic differentiation of stem and progenitor cells.[66-70] Recently, we have shown that biomineralized materials exhibiting dynamic dissolution-reprecipitation of CaP minerals can induce osteogenic differentiation of hMSCs, hESCs, and hiPSCs exclusively via the cues arising from the biomaterial – both *in vitro* and *in vivo*[18,71-74] (Figure 4.2a, b). More interestingly, the biomineralized matrices-induced osteogenic differentiation of hMSCs was observed even in the presence of media components that are known to induce adipogenic differentiation.[75] When implanted *in vivo*, these biomaterials recruited host cells to form vascularized bone tissues (subcutaneous[23] and posterolateral fusion[76]), even in the absence of any exogenous cells or osteoinductive growth factors (Figure 4.2c). These studies underscore the potential of such biomineralized materials to serve as a scaffold for *in situ* bone tissue engineering. Further analyses investigating the underlying molecular mechanism suggest that the CaP moieties of the mineralized materials induce osteogenic differentiation and inhibit adipogenic differentiation of stem cells through phosphate-adenosine triphosphate-adenosine metabolic signaling.[74,75] In addition, biomineralized materials are well established for their ability to adsorb and regulate growth factor signaling. For instance, CaP minerals are known to adsorb osteoinductive and angiogenic growth factors such as bone morphogenic proteins (BMPs) and VEGF,[77] suggesting their potential as delivery vehicles for such growth factors. An illustrative example was provided in a recent study by Lee *et al.*, in which multiple proteins were adsorbed and delivered from CaP multilayers in a controllable manner.[78] In addition to the inherent growth factor adsorption capacity, dissolution and reprecipitation of matrix-bound CaP can sequester and release osteoinductive growth factors. A recent work by Suarez-González *et al.* showed that release kinetics of BMP-2 was highly dictated by the dissolution of CaP moieties.[79] Dissolution of matrix-bound minerals leads to the release of adsorbed growth factor that could stimulate osteogenic differentiation of stem cells.

4.3 TUNING MATRIX STIFFNESS TO GUIDE CELL BEHAVIOR

In addition to the effects of biochemical cues, mechanical properties of the biomaterials are shown to influence a wide range of biological processes, including embryonic development,[80]

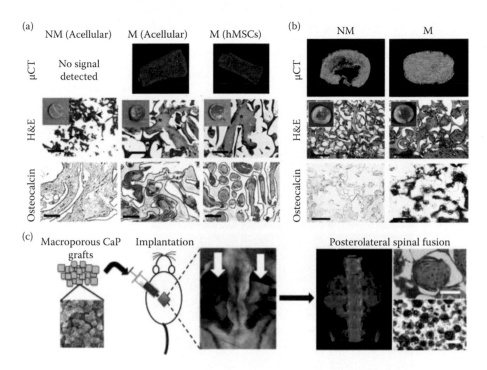

FIGURE 4.2 Biomineralized matrices-directed stem cell differentiation into osteoblasts and extraskeletal bone formation. (a) human embryonic stem cells (hESCs) on NM and M matrices and coverslips (CS) after *in vitro* culture. 3-D µCT images, H&E staining, and immunohistochemical staining for OCN of acellular NM and M and hMSC-laden M matrices and (b) hESC-laden NM and M matrices following *in vivo* subcutaneous implantation. Inset shows gross images. Scale bars indicate 50 µm and 100 µm for (a) and (b), respectively.[23,72] (c) Left, implantation of grafts in nude rats for posterolateral fusion; right, three-dimensional (3D) micro-computerized tomography (µCT) and transaxial cross-sectional images at 8 weeks after graft implantation; H&E and OCN staining reveal bone formation.[76] (a) Adapted from Phadke *et al.* (23), with permission; (b) adapted from Kang *et al.* (72), with permission, Copyright Royal Society of Chemistry, 2014; and (c) adapted from Shih *et al.* (76), with permission, Copyright 2015 Elsevier.

tissue homeostasis,[81] and disease pathogenesis.[6–8,82] The most often characterized and reported of the mechanical properties is matrix elasticity (or stiffness). Adhesion of cells to a material triggers signaling transduction cascades that allow for translation of extracellular mechanical cues into intracellular events.[83] The nature of these cascades varies with material elasticity, and controls several cell behaviors such as adhesion, spreading, migration, and cell shape through a variety of mechanosensors, which include integrins,[84–86] stretch-responsive ion channels,[87] and actomyosin cytoskeleton.[88] Signaling activities of focal adhesion kinase (FAK), Rho kinase (ROCK), and steroid receptor coactivator (SRC) family kinase are subsequently regulated to influence stem cell phenotypes.[89–91]

As such, hydrogels with different Young's modulus can be generated typically via varying cross-linking density,[92] precursor concentration,[93,94] or chemistry.[32,95,96] The results from studies investigating the effect of matrix stiffness on stem cell phenotype suggest

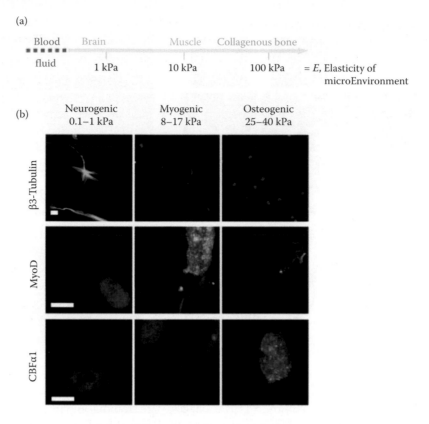

FIGURE 4.3 (a) Tissue stiffness: different tissues exhibit a range of stiffness, as measured by the elastic modulus, E. (b) The modulus of poly(acrylamide) substrates influences lineage-specific (neurogenic, myogenic or osteogenic) differentiation, as indicated by immunostaining for the appropriate markers (β3-tubulin, MyoD, and CBFα1, respectively, shown in green; cell nucleus in blue).[17] Adapted from Engler *et al.*, with permission, Copyright 2006 Elsevier.

that, in general, hydrogels with low (soft) and high (stiffer) Young's modulus regulate stem cell differentiation in unique ways with unique outcomes. For example, human MSCs were found to undergo neurogenesis on soft matrices ($E = 0.1$–$1\,kPa$), myogenesis on moderately stiff matrices ($E = 8$–$17\,kPa$), and osteogenesis on stiff matrices ($E = 25$–$40\,kPa$), respectively (Figure 4.3).[17] Other stem cell populations, including skeletal muscle stem cells,[97] neural progenitor cells,[98] and embryonic stem cells (ESCs),[99] have also been shown to exhibit substrate stiffness-dependent differentiation and function.

The effects of matrix stiffness have been further assessed in 3D cultures.[100–103] Similar to 2D cultures, MSCs were directed to differentiate into osteogenic or adipogenic lineage according to the substrate properties in which they were cultured; in this context, adhesion ligand presentation and local traction force were found to play pivotal roles.[100,101] As stem cells interact with their anchoring matrix through focal adhesion complexes, the integrin binding sites allow force balance transmission across the mechanical continuum of ECM-integrin-cytoskeleton, such that increased resistance to deformation in the matrix is correlated with strengthening of focal adhesions through activities of actomyosin network.

Such changes were found to have a significant effect on several kinase signaling pathways, including those of the FAK and SRC family,[91,104] as well as nuclear translocation of yes-associated protein,[105,106] all of which play key roles in stem cell fate determination.

Native ECM molecules such as collagen are nonlinear and viscoelastic in nature; however, the impact of nonlinear viscoelastic characteristics of ECM on cell functions remain relatively underexplored. This time-dependent, nonlinear characteristic of the ECM stems from the intricate interplays among cytoskeletal proteins, adhesion complexes, and extracellular environments,[107] further increasing the complexity of the mechanical environment. In a recent study, Chaudhuri et al. used 3D alginate hydrogels exhibiting stress relaxation properties to investigate the effects of nonlinear mechanical properties on stem cell behaviors.[20] Hydrogels with a faster rate of stress relaxation improved spreading, proliferation, and osteogenic differentiation of MSCs.[20] In a similar effort, Guvendiren and Burdick have used a methacrylated HA-based hydrogel with time-dependent matrix stiffening characteristics to probe the effects of dynamic mechanical properties on MSC differentiation.[108] Their results demonstrated that time-dependent changes in substrate stiffness evoked changes in stem cell phenotypes. In 2D culture, adipogenic differentiation of hMSCs was promoted with later matrix stiffening, while osteogenic differentiation was encouraged through earlier matrix stiffening.[108]

4.4 DESIGNING SYNTHETIC SUBSTRATE TO PROVIDE TOPOGRAPHICAL CUES

Paralleling the importance of ECM mechanics in regulating cellular functions, ECM proteins exhibit enormous nano/micrometer-scale features, which have been shown to profoundly impact cell signaling. For example, collagen fibers (diameter of several micrometers) are built from ordered collagen fibrils (diameter, 20–200 nm), which in turn are composed of triple helical collagen molecules (diameter, 1–10 nm).[109] Such hierarchical architectures and topographical features of native ECM (e.g., fibrillary structures) have been shown to contribute to various cellular functions.[110] Similarly, the basement membrane, a ubiquitous ECM component, displays unique nanotopographical characteristics that were found to modulate adhesion, migration, proliferation, and differentiation of the overlying epithelium.[111] Different approaches such as micropatterning, electrospinning, and photolithography have been used to create substrates with topographical features.[58,112–114] These advancements have enabled the investigation of cellular behaviors in response to a broad range of topographical features (e.g., lines, gratings, circles, and pillars) from single cell level to cell clusters in a systematic manner. Many of these techniques have been well reviewed by Théry.[114] In this section, we focus our discussion on the applications of substrate topography in regulating stem cell differentiation.

Development of cell substrates with topographical cues have been touted to provide reproducible and inexpensive systems for in vitro stem cell research.[115–119] For example, Ultra-Web™, a commercially available 3D nanofibrillar scaffold formed by depositing electrospun polyamine nanofibers onto the surface of the conventional cell culture plastics, was found to promote proliferation and self-renewal of ESCs compared to conventional tissue culture dishes.[117] In another study by Ji et al., substrates with highly ordered topographical features formed by organized arrangements of silica colloidal crystal microspheres demonstrated capacity for *in vitro* retention of pluripotency and restricted differentiation toward endoderm lineages.[118] A notable parallel can be found in topographically regulated MSC multipotency retentions on highly ordered arrays of nanopit surfaces.[119]

Substrates with topographical features have also been used to control *in vitro* differentiation of stem cells toward multiple lineages, including osteogenic,[120,121] myogenic,[122] and chondrogenic.[123] There is accumulating evidence that the size,[124] order,[120] and geometry[125] play critical roles in lineage differentiation of stem cells. For instance, hMSCs cultured on disordered nanopits were shown to undergo osteogenic differentiation in the absence of osteogenic induction media,[120] while MSCs maintained their multipotency on highly ordered nanopit surfaces.[119] Lovmand *et al.* utilized a combinatorial approach to identify optimal combinations of size, gap, and height of structures which enhance osteogenic differentiation by MC3T3-E1 (a preosteoblastic murine cell line).[126] Following the same approach, Markert *et al.* screened more than 500 topographically distinct micro-structured surfaces with murine ESCs, and they were able to assort the topographies supporting undifferentiated murine ESCs phenotypes and those inducing differentiation.[115] Topography at the nanoscale level has been found to change focal adhesion arrangement,[121,127] leading to changes in cytoskeletal configuration and mechanotransduction of the cells,[128,129] which results in differential gene expression and cell function, as mentioned in Section 3. In addition, the influence of nanotopographical features may be mediated through secondary effects, such as differences in protein adsorption due to the structural features of the substrate. While most studies involving topographical cues were focused on 2D cultures, pore architecture and size of scaffolds have been demonstrated to influence chondrogenic and osteogenic differentiation of stem cells in 3D cultures.[23,130]

4.5 CONCLUSIONS AND FUTURE PERSPECTIVES

The last two decades have witnessed a substantial paradigm shift in the design criteria of synthetic substrates with greater emphasis on integrating physicochemical principles of native tissue. Using these cell-instructive materials to guide stem cell functions (e.g., proliferation and differentiation of stem cells) remains a critical goal in the field of regenerative engineering to advance stem cell-based therapeutics and diagnostics. New approaches to functionalize common biomaterials with inductive capacities may help overcome cost barriers for effective stem cell expansion and differentiation, thereby enabling standardized manufacturing and scale-up processes. Novel strategies at the interface of materials science and stem cell biology will continue to be successfully applied to drive the development of regenerative engineering and allow for greater regulatory acceptance and clinical application of stem cell-based therapeutics.

REFERENCES

1. Fuchs, E.; Tumbar, T.; Guasch, G., Socializing with the neighbors: stem cells and their niche. *Cell* **2004**, *116* (6), 769–778.
2. Gumbiner, B. M., Cell adhesion: the molecular basis of tissue architecture and morphogenesis. *Cell* **1996**, *84* (3), 345–357.

3. Berrier, A. L.; Yamada, K. M., Cell-matrix adhesion. *J. Cell. Physiol.* **2007**, *213* (3), 565–573.
4. Palecek, S. P.; Loftus, J. C.; Ginsberg, M. H.; Lauffenburger, D. A.; Horwitz, A. F., Integrin-ligand binding properties govern cell migration speed through cell-substratum adhesiveness. *Nature* **1997**, *385* (6616), 537–540.
5. Nelson, C. M.; Bissell, M. J., Of extracellular matrix, scaffolds, and signaling: tissue architecture regulates development, homeostasis, and cancer. *Annu. Rev. Cell Dev. Biol.* **2006**, *22*, 287–309.
6. Friedl, P.; Alexander, S., Cancer invasion and the microenvironment: plasticity and reciprocity. *Cell* **2011**, *147* (5), 992–1009.
7. Lu, P.; Weaver, V. M.; Werb, Z., The extracellular matrix: a dynamic niche in cancer progression. *J. Cell Biol.* **2012**, *196* (4), 395–406.
8. Aung, A.; Seo, Y. N.; Lu, S.; Wang, Y.; Jamora, C.; del Alamo, J. C.; Varghese, S., 3D traction stresses activate protease-dependent invasion of cancer cells. *Biophys. J.* **2014**, *107* (11), 2528–2537.
9. Nakasaki, M.; Hwang, Y.; Xie, Y.; Kataria, S.; Gund, R.; Hajam, E. Y.; Samuel, R.; George, R.; Danda, D.; Paul, M., The matrix protein Fibulin-5 is at the interface of tissue stiffness and inflammation in fibrosis. *Nat. Commun.* **2015**, *6, 1–11.*
10. González-Díaz, E. C.; Varghese, S., Hydrogels as extracellular matrix analogs. *Gels* **2016**, *2* (3), 20.
11. Seale, N. M.; Varghese, S., Biomaterials for pluripotent stem cell engineering: from fate determination to vascularization. *J. Mater. Chem. B* **2016**, *4* (20), 3454–3463.
12. Drumheller, P. D.; Hubbell, J. A., Polymer networks with grafted cell adhesion peptides for highly biospecific cell adhesive substrates. *Anal. Biochem.* **1994**, *222* (2), 380–388.
13. Neff, J. A.; Tresco, P. A.; Caldwell, K. D., Surface modification for controlled studies of cell–ligand interactions. *Biomaterials* **1999**, *20* (23–24), 2377–2393.
14. Mosiewicz, K. A.; Kolb, L.; Van Der Vlies, A. J.; Martino, M. M.; Lienemann, P. S.; Hubbell, J. A.; Ehrbar, M.; Lutolf, M. P., In situ cell manipulation through enzymatic hydrogel photopatterning. *Nat. Mater.* **2013**, *12* (11), 1072–1078.
15. Sridhar, B. V.; Brock, J. L.; Silver, J. S.; Leight, J. L.; Randolph, M. A.; Anseth, K. S., Development of a cellularly degradable PEG hydrogel to promote articular cartilage extracellular matrix deposition. *Adv. Healthcare Mater.* **2015**, *4* (5), 702–713.
16. Varghese, S.; Hwang, N. S.; Canver, A. C.; Theprungsirikul, P.; Lin, D. W.; Elisseeff, J., Chondroitin sulfate based niches for chondrogenic differentiation of mesenchymal stem cells. *Matrix Biol.* **2008**, *27* (1), 12–21.
17. Engler, A. J.; Sen, S.; Sweeney, H. L.; Discher, D. E., Matrix elasticity directs stem cell lineage specification. *Cell* **2006**, *126* (4), 677–689.
18. Phadke, A.; Shih, Y.-R. V.; Varghese, S., Mineralized synthetic matrices as an instructive microenvironment for osteogenic differentiation of human mesenchymal stem cells. *Macromol. Biosci.* **2012**, *12* (8), 1022–1032.
19. Huebsch, N.; Lippens, E.; Lee, K.; Mehta, M.; Koshy, S. T.; Darnell, M. C.; Desai, R. M.; Madl, C. M.; Xu, M.; Zhao, X.; Chaudhuri, O.; Verbeke, C.; Kim, W. S.; Alim, K.; Mammoto, A.; Ingber, D. E.; Duda, G. N.; Mooney, D. J., Matrix elasticity of void-forming hydrogels controls transplanted-stem-cell-mediated bone formation. *Nat. Mater.* **2015**, *14* (12), 1269–1277.
20. Chaudhuri, O.; Gu, L.; Klumpers, D.; Darnell, M.; Bencherif, S. A.; Weaver, J. C.; Huebsch, N.; Lee, H. P.; Lippens, E.; Duda, G. N.; Mooney, D. J., Hydrogels with tunable stress relaxation regulate stem cell fate and activity. *Nat. Mater.* **2016**, *15* (3), 326–334.
21. Burdick, J. A.; Vunjak-Novakovic, G., Engineered microenvironments for controlled stem cell differentiation. *Tissue Eng. Part A* **2009**, *15* (2), 205–219.
22. Ayala, R.; Zhang, C.; Yang, D.; Hwang, Y.; Aung, A.; Shroff, S. S.; Arce, F. T.; Lal, R.; Arya, G.; Varghese, S., Engineering the cell–material interface for controlling stem cell adhesion, migration, and differentiation. *Biomaterials* **2011**, *32* (15), 3700–3711.

23. Phadke, A.; Hwang, Y.; Kim, S. H.; Kim, S. H.; Yamaguchi, T.; Masuda, K.; Varghese, S., Effect of scaffold microarchitecture on osteogenic differentiation of human mesenchymal stem cells. *Eur. Cells Mater.* **2013**, *25*, 114–129.

24. Dalby, M. J.; Gadegaard, N.; Oreffo, R. O., Harnessing nanotopography and integrin-matrix interactions to influence stem cell fate. *Nat. Mater.* **2014**, *13* (6), 558–569.

25. Lutolf, M.; Hubbell, J., Synthetic biomaterials as instructive extracellular microenvironments for morphogenesis in tissue engineering. *Nat. Biotech.* **2005**, *23* (1), 47–55.

26. Murphy, S. V.; Atala, A., 3D bioprinting of tissues and organs. *Nat. Biotech.* **2014**, *32* (8), 773–785.

27. Rodin, S.; Antonsson, L.; Niaudet, C.; Simonson, O. E.; Salmela, E.; Hansson, E. M.; Domogatskaya, A.; Xiao, Z.; Damdimopoulou, P.; Sheikhi, M.; Inzunza, J.; Nilsson, A. S.; Baker, D.; Kuiper, R.; Sun, Y.; Blennow, E.; Nordenskjold, M.; Grinnemo, K. H.; Kere, J.; Betsholtz, C.; Hovatta, O.; Tryggvason, K., Clonal culturing of human embryonic stem cells on laminin-521/E-cadherin matrix in defined and xeno-free environment. *Nat. Commun.* **2014**, *5*, 3195.

28. Kim, H. T.; Lee, K. I.; Kim, D. W.; Hwang, D. Y., An ECM-based culture system for the generation and maintenance of xeno-free human iPS cells. *Biomaterials* **2013**, *34* (4), 1041–1050.

29. Lutolf, M. P.; Hubbell, J. A., Synthesis and physicochemical characterization of end-linked poly(ethylene glycol)-co-peptide hydrogels formed by michael-type addition. *Biomacromolecules* **2003**, *4* (3), 713–722.

30. Klim, J. R.; Li, L.; Wrighton, P. J.; Piekarczyk, M. S.; Kiessling, L. L., A defined glycosaminoglycan-binding substratum for human pluripotent stem cells. *Nat. Methods* **2010**, *7* (12), 989–994.

31. Melkoumian, Z.; Weber, J. L.; Weber, D. M.; Fadeev, A. G.; Zhou, Y.; Dolley-Sonneville, P.; Yang, J.; Qiu, L.; Priest, C. A.; Shogbon, C.; Martin, A. W.; Nelson, J.; West, P.; Beltzer, J. P.; Pal, S.; Brandenberger, R., Synthetic peptide-acrylate surfaces for long-term self-renewal and cardiomyocyte differentiation of human embryonic stem cells. *Nat. Biotechnol.* **2010**, *28* (6), 606–610.

32. Mei, Y.; Saha, K.; Bogatyrev, S. R.; Yang, J.; Hook, A. L.; Ilke Kalcioglu, Z.; Cho, S.-W.; Mitalipova, M.; Pyzocha, N.; Rojas, F.; Van Vliet, K. J.; Davies, M. C.; Alexander, M. R.; Langer, R.; Jaenisch, R.; Anderson, D. G., Combinatorial development of biomaterials for clonal growth of human pluripotent stem cells. *Nat. Mater.* **2010**, *9* (9), 768–778.

33. Salinas, C. N.; Anseth, K. S., Decorin moieties tethered into PEG networks induce chondrogenesis of human mesenchymal stem cells. *J. Biomed. Mater. Res. A* **2009**, *90* (2), 456–464.

34. Hern, D. L.; Hubbell, J. A., Incorporation of adhesion peptides into nonadhesive hydrogels useful for tissue resurfacing. *J. Biomed. Mater. Res.* **1998**, *39* (2), 266–276.

35. Pierschbacher, M. D.; Ruoslahti, E., Influence of stereochemistry of the sequence Arg-Gly-Asp-Xaa on binding specificity in cell adhesion. *J. Biol. Chem.* **1987**, *262* (36), 17294–17298.

36. Santiago, L. Y.; Nowak, R. W.; Peter Rubin, J.; Marra, K. G., Peptide-surface modification of poly(caprolactone) with laminin-derived sequences for adipose-derived stem cell applications. *Biomaterials* **2006**, *27* (15), 2962–2969.

37. Lutolf, M.; Lauer-Fields, J.; Schmoekel, H.; Metters, A. T.; Weber, F.; Fields, G.; Hubbell, J. A., Synthetic matrix metalloproteinase-sensitive hydrogels for the conduction of tissue regeneration: engineering cell-invasion characteristics. *Proc. Natl. Acad. Sci.* **2003**, *100* (9), 5413–5418.

38. Burdick, J. A.; Chung, C.; Jia, X.; Randolph, M. A.; Langer, R., Controlled degradation and mechanical behavior of photopolymerized hyaluronic acid networks. *Biomacromolecules* **2005**, *6* (1), 386–391.

39. Bian, L.; Guvendiren, M.; Mauck, R. L.; Burdick, J. A., Hydrogels that mimic developmentally relevant matrix and N-cadherin interactions enhance MSC chondrogenesis. *Proc. Natl. Acad. Sci.* **2013**, *110* (25), 10117–10122.

40. Highley, C. B.; Prestwich, G. D.; Burdick, J. A., Recent advances in hyaluronic acid hydrogels for biomedical applications. *Curr. Opin. Biotechnol.* **2016**, *40*, 35–40.

41. Cai, S.; Liu, Y.; Zheng Shu, X.; Prestwich, G. D., Injectable glycosaminoglycan hydrogels for controlled release of human basic fibroblast growth factor. *Biomaterials* **2005**, *26* (30), 6054–6067.

42. Chang, C.-W.; Hwang, Y.; Brafman, D.; Hagan, T.; Phung, C.; Varghese, S., Engineering cell-material interfaces for long-term expansion of human pluripotent stem cells. *Biomaterials* **2013**, *34* (4), 912–921.

43. Sangaj, N.; Kyriakakis, P.; Yang, D.; Chang, C.-W.; Arya, G.; Varghese, S., Heparin mimicking polymer promotes myogenic differentiation of muscle progenitor cells. *Biomacromolecules* **2010**, *11* (12), 3294–3300.

44. Sakiyama-Elbert, S. E.; Hubbell, J. A., Development of fibrin derivatives for controlled release of heparin-binding growth factors. *J. Control Release* **2000**, *65* (3), 389–402.

45. Arai, T.; Busby, W., Jr.; Clemmons, D. R., Binding of insulin-like growth factor (IGF) I or II to IGF-binding protein-2 enables it to bind to heparin and extracellular matrix. *Endocrinology* **1996**, *137* (11), 4571–4575.

46. Benoit, D. S. W.; Anseth, K. S., Heparin functionalized PEG gels that modulate protein adsorption for hMSC adhesion and differentiation. *Acta Biomater.* **2005**, *1* (4), 461–470.

47. Rouet, V.; Hamma-Kourbali, Y.; Petit, E.; Panagopoulou, P.; Katsoris, P.; Barritault, D.; Caruelle, J.-P.; Courty, J., A synthetic glycosaminoglycan mimetic binds vascular endothelial growth factor and modulates angiogenesis. *J. Biol. Chem.* **2005**, *280* (38), 32792–32800.

48. Pike, D. B.; Cai, S.; Pomraning, K. R.; Firpo, M. A.; Fisher, R. J.; Shu, X. Z.; Prestwich, G. D.; Peattie, R. A., Heparin-regulated release of growth factors in vitro and angiogenic response in vivo to implanted hyaluronan hydrogels containing VEGF and bFGF. *Biomaterials* **2006**, *27* (30), 5242–5251.

49. Saksela, O.; Moscatelli, D.; Sommer, A.; Rifkin, D. B., Endothelial cell-derived heparan sulfate binds basic fibroblast growth factor and protects it from proteolytic degradation. *J. Cell Biol.* **1988**, *107* (2), 743–751.

50. Prokoph, S.; Chavakis, E.; Levental, K. R.; Zieris, A.; Freudenberg, U.; Dimmeler, S.; Werner, C., Sustained delivery of SDF-1alpha from heparin-based hydrogels to attract circulating pro-angiogenic cells. *Biomaterials* **2012**, *33* (19), 4792–4800.

51. Seto, S. P.; Miller, T.; Temenoff, J. S., Effect of selective heparin desulfation on preservation of bone morphogenetic protein-2 bioactivity after thermal stress. *Bioconjug. Chem.* **2015**, *26* (2), 286–293.

52. Kabra, H.; Hwang, Y.; Lim, H. L.; Kar, M.; Arya, G.; Varghese, S., Biomimetic material-assisted delivery of human embryonic stem cell derivatives for enhanced in vivo survival and engraftment. *ACS Biomater. Sci. Eng.* **2015**, *1* (1), 7–12.

53. Jha, A. K.; Tharp, K. M.; Ye, J.; Santiago-Ortiz, J. L.; Jackson, W. M.; Stahl, A.; Schaffer, D. V.; Yeghiazarians, Y.; Healy, K. E., Enhanced survival and engraftment of transplanted stem cells using growth factor sequestering hydrogels. *Biomaterials* **2015**, *47*, 1–12.

54. Hudalla, G. A.; Koepsel, J. T.; Murphy, W. L., Surfaces that sequester serum-borne heparin amplify growth factor activity. *Adv. Mater.* **2011**, *23* (45), 5415–5418.

55. Curran, J. M.; Chen, R.; Hunt, J. A., The guidance of human mesenchymal stem cell differentiation in vitro by controlled modifications to the cell substrate. *Biomaterials* **2006**, *27* (27), 4783–4793.

56. Keselowsky, B. G.; Collard, D. M.; García, A. J., Integrin binding specificity regulates biomaterial surface chemistry effects on cell differentiation. *Proc. Natl. Acad. Sci. U. S. A.* **2005**, *102* (17), 5953–5957.

57. Keselowsky, B. G.; Collard, D. M.; García, A. J., Surface chemistry modulates focal adhesion composition and signaling through changes in integrin binding. *Biomaterials* **2004**, *25* (28), 5947–5954.

58. Benoit, D. S. W.; Schwartz, M. P.; Durney, A. R.; Anseth, K. S., Small functional groups for controlled differentiation of hydrogel-encapsulated human mesenchymal stem cells. *Nat. Mater.* **2008**, *7* (10), 816–823.

59. Mann, S., Molecular tectonics in biomineralization and biomimetic materials chemistry. *Nature* **1993**, *365* (6446), 499–505.

60. Suárez-González, D.; Barnhart, K.; Saito, E.; Vanderby, R., Jr.; Hollister, S. J.; Murphy, W. L., Controlled nucleation of hydroxyapatite on alginate scaffolds for stem cell-based bone tissue engineering. *J. Biomed. Mater. Res. A* **2010**, *95* (1), 222–234.

61. Phadke, A.; Zhang, C.; Hwang, Y.; Vecchio, K.; Varghese, S., Templated mineralization of synthetic hydrogels for bone-like composite materials: role of matrix hydrophobicity. *Biomacromolecules* **2010**, *11* (8), 2060–2068.

62. Murphy, W. L.; Mooney, D. J., Bioinspired growth of crystalline carbonate apatite on biodegradable polymer substrata. *J. Am. Chem. Soc.* **2002**, *124* (9), 1910–1917.

63. Song, J.; Saiz, E.; Bertozzi, C. R., A new approach to mineralization of biocompatible hydrogel scaffolds: an efficient process toward 3-dimensional bonelike composites. *J. Am. Chem. Soc.* **2003**, *125* (5), 1236–1243.

64. Sasaki, S.; Yataki, K.; Maeda, H., Effect of the hydrophobicity of chain on Ca^{2+} binding to ionic gels. *Langmuir* **1998**, *14* (4), 796–799.

65. Varghese, S.; Lele, A. K.; Srinivas, D.; Mashelkar, R. A., Role of hydrophobicity on structure of polymer–metal complexes. *J. Phys. Chem. B* **2001**, *105* (23), 5368–5373.

66. Grayson, W. L.; Bhumiratana, S.; Grace Chao, P. H.; Hung, C. T.; Vunjak-Novakovic, G., Spatial regulation of human mesenchymal stem cell differentiation in engineered osteochondral constructs: effects of pre-differentiation, soluble factors and medium perfusion. *Osteoarthritis Cartilage* **2010**, *18* (5), 714–723.

67. ter Brugge, P. J.; Wolke, J. G. C.; Jansen, J. A., Effect of calcium phosphate coating crystallinity and implant surface roughness on differentiation of rat bone marrow cells. *J. Biomed. Mater. Res.* **2002**, *60* (1), 70–78.

68. Yuan, H.; Fernandes, H.; Habibovic, P.; de Boer, J.; Barradas, A. M. C.; de Ruiter, A.; Walsh, W. R.; van Blitterswijk, C. A.; de Bruijn, J. D., Osteoinductive ceramics as a synthetic alternative to autologous bone grafting. *Proc. Natl. Acad. Sci. U. S. A.* **2010**, *107* (31), 13614–13619.

69. Reichert, J. C.; Cipitria, A.; Epari, D. R.; Saifzadeh, S.; Krishnakanth, P.; Berner, A.; Woodruff, M. A.; Schell, H.; Mehta, M.; Schuetz, M. A.; Duda, G. N.; Hutmacher, D. W., A tissue engineering solution for segmental defect regeneration in load-bearing long bones. *Sci. Transl. Med.* **2012**, *4* (141), 141ra93.

70. Hwang, N. S.; Varghese, S.; Lee, H. J.; Zhang, Z.; Elisseeff, J., Biomaterials directed in vivo osteogenic differentiation of mesenchymal cells derived from human embryonic stem cells. *Tissue Eng. Part A* **2013**, *19* (15–16), 1723–1732.

71. Kang, H.; Shih, Y.-R. V.; Hwang, Y.; Wen, C.; Rao, V.; Seo, T.; Varghese, S., Mineralized gelatin methacrylate-based matrices induce osteogenic differentiation of human induced pluripotent stem cells. *Acta Biomater.* **2014**, *10* (12), 4961–4970.

72. Kang, H.; Wen, C.; Hwang, Y.; Shih, Y.-R. V.; Kar, M.; Seo, S. W.; Varghese, S., Biomineralized matrix-assisted osteogenic differentiation of human embryonic stem cells. *J. Mater. Chem. B Mater. Biol. Med.* **2014**, *2* (34), 5676–5688.

73. Wen, C.; Kang, H.; Shih, Y.-R. V.; Hwang, Y.; Varghese, S., In vivo comparison of biomineralized scaffold-directed osteogenic differentiation of human embryonic and mesenchymal stem cells. *Drug Deliv. Transl. Res.* **2016**, *6* (2), 121–131.

74. Shih, Y.-R. V.; Hwang, Y.; Phadke, A.; Kang, H.; Hwang, N. S.; Caro, E. J.; Nguyen, S.; Siu, M.; Theodorakis, E. A.; Gianneschi, N. C.; Vecchio, K. S.; Chien, S.; Lee, O. K.; Varghese, S., Calcium phosphate-bearing matrices induce osteogenic differentiation of stem cells through adenosine signaling. *Proc. Natl. Acad. Sci. U. S. A.* **2014**, *111* (3), 990–995.

75. Kang, H.; Shih, Y. R.; Varghese, S., Biomineralized matrices dominate soluble cues to direct osteogenic differentiation of human mesenchymal stem cells through adenosine signaling. *Biomacromolecules* **2015**, *16* (3), 1050–1061.

76. Shih, Y.-R.; Phadke, A.; Yamaguchi, T.; Kang, H.; Inoue, N.; Masuda, K.; Varghese, S., Synthetic bone mimetic matrix-mediated in situ bone tissue formation through host cell recruitment. *Acta Biomater.* **2015**, *19*, 1–9.

77. Lode, A.; Wolf-Brandstetter, C.; Reinstorf, A.; Bernhardt, A.; König, U.; Pompe, W.; Gelinsky, M., Calcium phosphate bone cements, functionalized with VEGF: release kinetics and biological activity. *J. Biomed. Mater. Res. Part A* **2007**, *81* (2), 474–483.

78. Lee, J. S.; Suarez-González, D.; Murphy, W. L., Mineral coatings for temporally controlled delivery of multiple proteins. *Adv. Mater.* **2011**, *23* (37), 4279–4284.

79. Suarez-González, D.; Barnhart, K.; Migneco, F.; Flanagan, C.; Hollister, S. J.; Murphy, W. L., Controllable mineral coatings on PCL scaffolds as carriers for growth factor release. *Biomaterials* **2012**, *33* (2), 713–721.

80. Mammoto, T.; Ingber, D. E., Mechanical control of tissue and organ development. *Development* **2010**, *137* (9), 1407–1420.

81. Wozniak, M. A.; Chen, C. S., Mechanotransduction in development: a growing role for contractility. *Nat. Rev. Mol. Cell Biol.* **2009**, *10* (1), 34–43.

82. Paszek, M. J.; Weaver, V. M., The tension mounts: mechanics meets morphogenesis and malignancy. *J. Mammary Gland Biol. Neoplasia* **2004**, *9* (4), 325–342.

83. Ingber, D. E., Cellular mechanotransduction: putting all the pieces together again. *FASEB J.* **2006**, *20* (7), 811–827.

84. Balaban, N. Q.; Schwarz, U. S.; Riveline, D.; Goichberg, P.; Tzur, G.; Sabanay, I.; Mahalu, D.; Safran, S.; Bershadsky, A.; Addadi, L.; Geiger, B., Force and focal adhesion assembly: a close relationship studied using elastic micropatterned substrates. *Nat. Cell Biol.* **2001**, *3* (5), 466–472.

85. Galbraith, C. G.; Yamada, K. M.; Sheetz, M. P., The relationship between force and focal complex development. *J. Cell Biol.* **2002**, *159* (4), 695–705.

86. Meyer, C. J.; Alenghat, F. J.; Rim, P.; Fong, J. H.; Fabry, B.; Ingber, D. E., Mechanical control of cyclic AMP signalling and gene transcription through integrins. *Nat. Cell Biol.* **2000**, *2* (9), 666–668.

87. Martinac, B., Mechanosensitive ion channels: molecules of mechanotransduction. *J. Cell Sci.* **2004**, *117* (Pt 12), 2449–2460.

88. Wang, N.; Butler, J. P.; Ingber, D. E., Mechanotransduction across the cell surface and through the cytoskeleton. *Science* **1993**, *260* (5111), 1124–1127.

89. Shih, Y.-R. V.; Tseng, K.-F.; Lai, H.-Y.; Lin, C.-H.; Lee, O. K., Matrix stiffness regulation of integrin-mediated mechanotransduction during osteogenic differentiation of human mesenchymal stem cells. *J. Bone Miner. Res.* **2011**, *26* (4), 730–738.

90. Fu, J.; Wang, Y.-K.; Yang, M. T.; Desai, R. A.; Yu, X.; Liu, Z.; Chen, C. S., Mechanical regulation of cell function with geometrically modulated elastomeric substrates. *Nat. Methods* **2010**, *7* (9), 733–736.

91. Schlaepfer, D. D.; Hauck, C. R.; Sieg, D. J., Signaling through focal adhesion kinase. *Prog. Biophys. Mol. Biol.* **1999**, *71* (3–4), 435–478.

92. Kim, I. L.; Khetan, S.; Baker, B. M.; Chen, C. S.; Burdick, J. A., Fibrous hyaluronic acid hydrogels that direct MSC chondrogenesis through mechanical and adhesive cues. *Biomaterials* **2013**, *34* (22), 5571–5580.

93. Marklein, R. A.; Burdick, J. A., Spatially controlled hydrogel mechanics to modulate stem cell interactions. *Soft Matter* **2009**, *6* (1), 136–143.

94. Lin, S.; Sangaj, N.; Razafiarison, T.; Zhang, C.; Varghese, S., Influence of physical properties of biomaterials on cellular behavior. *Pharm. Res.* **2011**, *28* (6), 1422–1430.

95. Awad, H. A.; Wickham, M. Q.; Leddy, H. A.; Gimble, J. M.; Guilak, F., Chondrogenic differentiation of adipose-derived adult stem cells in agarose, alginate, and gelatin scaffolds. *Biomaterials* **2004**, *25* (16), 3211–3222.

96. Zhang, C.; Aung, A.; Liao, L.; Varghese, S., A novel single precursor-based biodegradable hydrogel with enhanced mechanical properties. *Soft Matter.* **2009**, *5* (20), 3831–3834.

97. Gilbert, P. M.; Havenstrite, K. L.; Magnusson, K. E. G.; Sacco, A.; Leonardi, N. A.; Kraft, P.; Nguyen, N. K.; Thrun, S.; Lutolf, M. P.; Blau, H. M., Substrate elasticity regulates skeletal muscle stem cell self-renewal in culture. *Science* **2010**, *329* (5995), 1078–1081.

98. Saha, K.; Keung, A. J.; Irwin, E. F.; Li, Y.; Little, L.; Schaffer, D. V.; Healy, K. E., Substrate modulus directs neural stem cell behavior. *Biophys. J.* **2008**, *95* (9), 4426–4438.

99. Evans, N. D.; Minelli, C.; Gentleman, E.; LaPointe, V.; Patankar, S. N.; Kallivretaki, M.; Chen, X.; Roberts, C. J.; Stevens, M. M., Substrate stiffness affects early differentiation events in embryonic stem cells. *Eur. Cell. Mater.* **2009**, *18*, 1–13; discussion 13–4.

100. Huebsch, N.; Arany, P. R.; Mao, A. S.; Shvartsman, D.; Ali, O. A.; Bencherif, S. A.; Rivera-Feliciano, J.; Mooney, D. J., Harnessing traction-mediated manipulation of the cell-matrix interface to control stem cell fate. *Nat. Mater.* **2010**, *9* (6), 518–526.

101. Khetan, S.; Guvendiren, M.; Legant, W. R.; Cohen, D. M.; Chen, C. S.; Burdick, J. A., Degradation-mediated cellular traction directs stem cell fate in covalently crosslinked three-dimensional hydrogels. *Nat. Mater.* **2013**, *12* (5), 458–465.

102. Her, G. J.; Wu, H.-C.; Chen, M.-H.; Chen, M.-Y.; Chang, S.-C.; Wang, T.-W., Control of three-dimensional substrate stiffness to manipulate mesenchymal stem cell fate toward neuronal or glial lineages. *Acta Biomater.* **2013**, *9* (2), 5170–5180.

103. Kloxin, A. M.; Kasko, A. M.; Salinas, C. N.; Anseth, K. S., Photodegradable hydrogels for dynamic tuning of physical and chemical properties. *Science* **2009**, *324* (5923), 59–63.

104. Salasznyk, R. M.; Klees, R. F.; Boskey, A.; Plopper, G. E., Activation of FAK is necessary for the osteogenic differentiation of human mesenchymal stem cells on laminin-5. *J. Cell Biochem.* **2007**, *100* (2), 499–514.

105. Dupont, S.; Morsut, L.; Aragona, M.; Enzo, E.; Giulitti, S.; Cordenonsi, M.; Zanconato, F.; Le Digabel, J.; Forcato, M.; Bicciato, S.; Elvassore, N.; Piccolo, S., Role of YAP/TAZ in mechanotransduction. *Nature* **2011**, *474* (7350), 179–183.

106. Lian, I.; Kim, J.; Okazawa, H.; Zhao, J.; Zhao, B.; Yu, J.; Chinnaiyan, A.; Israel, M. A.; Goldstein, L. S.; Abujarour, R.; Ding, S.; Guan, K. L., The role of YAP transcription coactivator in regulating stem cell self-renewal and differentiation. *Genes Dev.* **2010**, *24* (11), 1106–1118.

107. Storm, C.; Pastore, J. J.; MacKintosh, F. C.; Lubensky, T. C.; Janmey, P. A., Nonlinear elasticity in biological gels. *Nature* **2005**, *435* (7039), 191–194.

108. Guvendiren, M.; Burdick, J. A., Stiffening hydrogels to probe short- and long-term cellular responses to dynamic mechanics. *Nat. Commun.* **2012**, *3*, 792.

109. Birk, D. E.; Zycband, E. I.; Winkelmann, D. A.; Trelstad, R. L., Collagen fibrillogenesis in situ: fibril segments are intermediates in matrix assembly. *Proc. Natl. Acad. Sci. U. S. A.* **1989**, *86* (12), 4549–4553.

110. Stevens, M. M.; George, J. H., Exploring and engineering the cell surface interface. *Science* **2005**, *310* (5751), 1135–1138.

111. Juliano, R. L.; Haskill, S., Signal transduction from the extracellular matrix. *J. Cell Biol.* **1993**, *120* (3), 577–585.

112. Hahn, M. S.; Miller, J. S.; West, J. L., Three-dimensional biochemical and biomechanical patterning of hydrogels for guiding cell behavior. *Adv. Mater.* **2006**, *18* (20), 2679–2684.

113. DeForest, C. A.; Tirrell, D. A., A photoreversible protein-patterning approach for guiding stem cell fate in three-dimensional gels. *Nat. Mater.* **2015**, *14* (5), 523–531.

114. Théry, M., Micropatterning as a tool to decipher cell morphogenesis and functions. *J. Cell Sci.* **2010**, *123* (Pt 24), 4201–4213.

115. Markert, L. D. a.; Lovmand, J.; Foss, M.; Lauridsen, R. H.; Lovmand, M.; Füchtbauer, E.-M.; Füchtbauer, A.; Wertz, K.; Besenbacher, F.; Pedersen, F. S.; Duch, M., Identification of distinct topographical surface microstructures favoring either undifferentiated expansion or differentiation of murine embryonic stem cells. *Stem Cells Dev.* **2009**, *18* (9), 1331–1342.

116. Guvendiren, M.; Burdick, J. A., The control of stem cell morphology and differentiation by hydrogel surface wrinkles. *Biomaterials* **2010**, *31* (25), 6511–6518.

117. Nur-E-Kamal, A.; Ahmed, I.; Kamal, J.; Schindler, M.; Meiners, S., Three-dimensional nanofibrillar surfaces promote self-renewal in mouse embryonic stem cells. *Stem Cells* **2006**, *24* (2), 426–433.

118. Ji, L.; LaPointe, V. L. S.; Evans, N. D.; Stevens, M. M., Changes in embryonic stem cell colony morphology and early differentiation markers driven by colloidal crystal topographical cues. *Eur. Cell. Mater.* **2012**, *23*, 135–146.

119. McMurray, R. J.; Gadegaard, N.; Tsimbouri, P. M.; Burgess, K. V.; McNamara, L. E.; Tare, R.; Murawski, K.; Kingham, E.; Oreffo, R. O. C.; Dalby, M. J., Nanoscale surfaces for the long-term maintenance of mesenchymal stem cell phenotype and multipotency. *Nat. Mater.* **2011**, *10* (8), 637–644.

120. Dalby, M. J.; Gadegaard, N.; Tare, R.; Andar, A.; Riehle, M. O.; Herzyk, P.; Wilkinson, C. D. W.; Oreffo, R. O. C., The control of human mesenchymal cell differentiation using nanoscale symmetry and disorder. *Nat. Mater.* **2007**, *6* (12), 997–1003.

121. Oh, S.; Brammer, K. S.; Li, Y. S. J.; Teng, D.; Engler, A. J.; Chien, S.; Jin, S., Stem cell fate dictated solely by altered nanotube dimension. *Proc. Natl. Acad. Sci. U. S. A.* **2009**, *106* (7), 2130–2135.

122. Dang, J. M.; Leong, K. W., Myogenic induction of aligned mesenchymal stem cell sheets by culture on thermally responsive electrospun nanofibers. *Adv. Mater.* **2007**, *19* (19), 2775–2779.

123. Muraglia, A.; Cancedda, R.; Quarto, R., Clonal mesenchymal progenitors from human bone marrow differentiate in vitro according to a hierarchical model. *J. Cell Sci.* **2000**, *113 (Pt 7)*, 1161–1166.

124. Yim, E. K. F.; Pang, S. W.; Leong, K. W., Synthetic nanostructures inducing differentiation of human mesenchymal stem cells into neuronal lineage. *Exp. Cell Res.* **2007**, *313* (9), 1820–1829.

125. Ankam, S.; Suryana, M.; Chan, L. Y.; Moe, A. A. K.; Teo, B. K. K.; Law, J. B. K.; Sheetz, M. P.; Low, H. Y.; Yim, E. K. F., Substrate topography and size determine the fate of human embryonic stem cells to neuronal or glial lineage. *Acta Biomater.* **2013**, *9* (1), 4535–4545.

126. Lovmand, J.; Justesen, J.; Foss, M.; Lauridsen, R. H.; Lovmand, M.; Modin, C.; Besenbacher, F.; Pedersen, F. S.; Duch, M., The use of combinatorial topographical libraries for the screening of enhanced osteogenic expression and mineralization. *Biomaterials* **2009**, *30* (11), 2015–2022.

127. Chen, W.; Villa-Diaz, L. G.; Sun, Y.; Weng, S.; Kim, J. K.; Lam, R. H. W.; Han, L.; Fan, R.; Krebsbach, P. H.; Fu, J., Nanotopography influences adhesion, spreading, and self-renewal of human embryonic stem cells. *ACS Nano* **2012**, *6* (5), 4094–4103.

128. Arnold, M.; Cavalcanti-Adam, E. A.; Glass, R.; Blummel, J.; Eck, W.; Kantlehner, M.; Kessler, H.; Spatz, J. P., Activation of integrin function by nanopatterned adhesive interfaces. *Chemphyschem* **2004**, *5* (3), 383–388.

129. Gerecht, S.; Bettinger, C. J.; Zhang, Z.; Borenstein, J. T.; Vunjak-Novakovic, G.; Langer, R., The effect of actin disrupting agents on contact guidance of human embryonic stem cells. *Biomaterials* **2007**, *28* (28), 4068–4077.

130. Levingstone, T. J.; Matsiko, A.; Dickson, G. R.; O'Brien, F. J.; Gleeson, J. P., A biomimetic multi-layered collagen-based scaffold for osteochondral repair. *Acta Biomater.* **2014**, *10* (5), 1996–2004.

CHAPTER 5

Bovine Tissue-Scaffold Interface Facilitates *in vivo* Evaluation of Tissue-Engineered Injectable Devices for Breast Tissue Reconstruction

Cheryl T. Gomillion and Karen J. L. Burg

University of Georgia

Steven E. Ellis[*]

National Science Foundation

CONTENTS

---

[*] The views expressed in this chapter do not necessarily reflect those of the National Science Foundation or the United States Government.

5.1 INTRODUCTION

Breast reconstruction procedures are commonly performed following tumor removal to restore the appearance of the breast to its normal contour and size. Numerous breast reconstruction procedures, including placement of breast implants and autologous tissue transfers, for example, are performed each year in the United States. Many complications associated with frequently used methods for breast reconstruction exist (Gomillion *et al.*, 2007). Specifically, the use of autologous fat tissue transplantation as a means for breast reconstruction has been largely unsuccessful due to resorption of transplanted adipose tissue over time (Patrick, 2004; Simonacci *et al.*, 2016). Because breast tissue is largely composed of adipose tissue, the development of breast tissue engineering strategies focused on regeneration of adipose tissue is of great interest to researchers who realize the need for alternate reconstruction methods. The ability to successfully reconstruct breast tissue using tissue engineering methods, however, has been limited to date because of an inability to produce large amounts of engineered adipose tissue that retain volume and remain viable over time (Choi *et al.*, 2010; Patrick, 2000, 2001; Patrick *et al.*, 1998; Renneker and Cutler, 1952). Only recently has one reported study described minimal success attempting to reconstruct the human breast post mastectomy using large volumes of engineered adipose tissue. However, the method described in this proof-of-concept study involved use of a nondegradable acrylic chamber within the patient's chest wall, which required removal several months post implantation, further contributing to the patient's strain and expense (Morrison *et al.*, 2016).

The development of a clinically translatable method of engineering adipose tissue for breast reconstruction requires the investigation of several components. For the engineering of any tissue to be successful, attention must be paid to all key aspects of the tissue engineering process, including the cell source, scaffold (also termed "construct") material, cellular environment, and means of device delivery (Gomillion and Burg, 2006, 2011). Adipose-derived stem cells, preadipocytes, and mature adipocytes have been suggested for use in adipose tissue engineering systems; however, the uncertainty behind the mechanisms of adipogenesis *in vitro* has limited progress with reconstructing tissue (Ailhaud *et al.*, 1992; Beahm *et al.*, 2003; De Ugarte *et al.*, 2003; Hemmrich *et al.*, 2005; Patrick, 2000). The materials used for constructing the scaffolds, whether implanted or injected, must possess several essential properties. These materials should be biocompatible, biodegradable, nontoxic, easily produced, easily managed during surgical procedures, and should guide the migration and proliferation of cells (Alhadlaq *et al.*, 2005; Chen *et al.*, 2002; Fuchs *et al.*, 2001; Katz *et al.*, 1999; Walgenbach *et al.*, 2001). In addition, to allow adequate cellular growth, the construct formed should be porous to allow binding sites for cellular ingrowth and the permeation of nutrients and waste products in and out of the construct (Walgenbach *et al.*, 2001).

When selecting a material for use as scaffolding in adipose tissue engineering, several variables must be considered. Scaffold selection depends on the physical, mechanical, and chemical properties of the materials (Alhadlaq *et al.*, 2005). Because the tissue that is being reconstructed is a "soft" tissue, a scaffold material that imparts a natural feel, comparable to the native tissue, is ideal, particularly for restoration of breast tissue in women (Beahm *et al.*, 2003; Halberstadt *et al.*, 2002; Rowley *et al.*, 1999; Young and Christman, 2012). Additionally, adipocytes and preadipocytes are anchorage-dependent cells, meaning that they must adhere to a biomaterial of sufficient stiffness in order for proliferation and differentiation to occur (Atala and Lanza, 2002; Patrick, 2000, 2001). Accordingly, researchers have investigated modifying the surface and porosity of traditional "bulk" scaffolds to encourage cellular attachment while allowing the diffusion of nutrients and vascularization within a construct (Beahm *et al.*, 2003; Burg and Shalaby, 1999).

Since first disclosing the concept of a composite injectable in 1999 (Burg, 2000), our research has been directed toward the development of a minimally invasive device for breast tissue reconstruction. The injectable composite system incorporates biodegradable, injectable microcarrier beads of tunable modulus on which anchorage-dependent cells may be seeded, and a hydrogel delivery medium to stimulate regeneration of host adipose cells to fill soft tissue voids in the breast (Burg, 2006; Gomillion and Burg, 2000). The basic concept envisioned for this method is described as follows: patient cells are seeded on absorbable beads of an injectable size (diameter smaller than the gauge of a selected needle) to form cell carriers that would then be mixed with a degradable hydrogel carrier. The resulting construct could then be delivered to a defect site in a patient through a syringe injection. Hence, we first proposed the use of injectable beads as a scaffold material to allow a minimally invasive procedure that would eliminate the need for subsequent traumatic surgeries for breast cancer patients, effectively reducing the patient's pain, scarring, recovery time, and expense. These injectable scaffolds could be manufactured to be softer than typical polymer scaffolds and, because of their injectable nature, would be able to conform to various shapes to fill defect sites. Because of their smaller individual volume, they have the potential to restore the texture and volume of natural breast tissue more effectively than larger scaffolds, such as polymer sponges and foams, because they would facilitate the infiltration of healthy tissue (Burg and Boland, 2003; Choi *et al.*, 2005; McGlohorn *et al.*, 2003).

To fully investigate the potential of the injectable composite, an applicable large animal model in which these systems may be evaluated must also be determined (Lanza *et al.*, 2000; Patrick, 2004; Patrick *et al.*, 2008). Previous studies have shown the ability of researchers to regenerate adipose tissue to repair small-volume soft tissue defects in smaller animals, including rats and nude mice. Studies have also demonstrated the ability to induce adipose tissue formation within the subcutaneous space of sheep (Halberstadt *et al.*, 2002); however, further investigation of this technology within a large animal that has biological and size characteristics comparable to that of humans and specifically facilitates increased animal welfare is warranted (Gomillion *et al.*, 2007). It has been demonstrated previously, comparing implants in rodents to those in humans, that the mass ratio of implant to biological system is extremely important in determining implant biocompatibility. Also, cows have an exceptionally low incidence of mammary tumors (Bierła *et al.*, 2012; Borena *et al.*, 2013; Capuco and Ellis, 2005; Ford *et al.*, 1989; Petrites-Murphy, 1992); hence, they provide an interesting model which can be studied to understand the protectant nature.

The bovine mammary gland consists of comparable anatomical structures and tissue types as that of the normal human breast (Akers, 2002). A histological evaluation reveals that bovine mammary tissue is more similar to that of humans than is mammary tissue of traditional animal models such as mice and rats. The ductal structures in humans and dairy cattle are surrounded by relatively dense stromal tissue (Capuco and Ellis, 2005; Rowson *et al.*, 2012; Russo *et al.*, 2001), unlike the ducts in murine mammary glands, which are nearly completely enclosed by adipocytes (Lee *et al.*, 2003). More importantly, in addition to the structural and anatomical similarities that exist between human and bovine tissue, conserved synteny between the human and bovine genome has been well defined through comparative mapping and chromosome painting studies (Band *et al.*, 2000, Solinas-Toldo *et al.*, 1995, Threadgill and Womack, 1990, Threadgill *et al.*, 1990, Womack and Kata, 1995). Furthermore, studies have also demonstrated that cytokines found in the bovine mammary gland, such as interleukin (IL)-1α, IL-1β, IL-2, IL8, IL-12, interferon-γ, and tumor necrosis factor-α, have a high level of homology (>80% in some instances) with specific human proteins (Alluwaimi, 2004).

We, therefore, performed this proof-of-concept study to evaluate the feasibility of injectable tissue-engineered devices using a bovine model to assess their *in vivo* biocompatibility. We hypothesized that an injectable tissue-engineered device, in contrast to the traditional bulk implant, would allow infiltration of host tissue throughout its volume, facilitating growth of new adipose tissue *in vivo*. The injectable tissue-engineered devices were implanted intradermally, not in the mammary gland, to determine if the cells that were implanted in our device had the capacity for stimulating adipose tissue formation and to better distinguish new adipose tissue from native adipose tissue post implantation since adipose tissue is not normally found within the skin. This location was also selected to provide superior containment of the material injected and, therefore, ease of later identification and harvest. This study is the first reported use of a bovine model for a tissue engineering system of this kind, thus testing the potential of an alternate large animal model for preclinical testing of regenerative therapies.

5.2 MATERIALS AND METHODS

5.2.1 Scaffold Fabrication

CultiSpher-S Gelatin (type A porcine gelatin) microcarriers (diameter, 130–380 µm), purchased in dehydrated form (Percell Biolytica, Åstorp, Sweden), were hydrated under sterile conditions in calcium-free and magnesium-free phosphate buffered saline (PBS) (Sigma, St. Louis, MO). Poly-L-lactide (PL) (Cargill, Minneapolis, MN) beads were fabricated using a single-emulsion process (Brown *et al.*, 2005). A 20% w/v polymer solution was prepared by dissolving the as-received PL pellets (as-received MW = 195 ± 2 kDa) in dichloromethane (Mallinckrodt, Phillipsburg, NJ) (Thomas, 2011. The beads were formed by injecting the polymer solution from a 20-mL syringe (Becton Dickinson, Franklin Lakes, NJ), equipped with a 16-gauge needle (Becton Dickinson) into a continuously stirred solution of 0.3% w/v poly(vinyl alcohol) (Sigma). The beads were then washed in a 2% v/v solution of isopropanol (VWR, West Chester, PA), dried, sieved using stainless-steel strainers to sort by size (diameter, 250–425 µm), and stored under house vacuum until use. The PL beads were soaked in 70% ethanol (Pharmco-Aaper, Shelbyville, KY), and were then soaked in fresh culture medium immediately before use (post processing MW = 175 ± 4 kDa) (Thomas, 2011).

5.2.2 Adipose Tissue Retrieval and Cell Isolation

All experimental procedures were performed in accordance with a protocol approved by the Clemson University Institutional Animal Care and Use Committee. Subcutaneous adipose tissue samples were obtained from three Holstein heifers. Following intravenous (i.v.) administration of acepromazine (Vedco, Inc., St. Joseph, MO), the left tail-head region at the rear of each heifer was shaved and washed with Betadine® (Purdue Frederick Co., Stamford, CT). Lidocaine (Vedco, Inc.) was locally administered at the shaved tail-head region, and subcutaneous adipose tissue samples (at least 4 g pcr heifer) were excised from the left tail-head region of each heifer by making an "S"-shaped incision with a disposable scalpel (Becton Dickinson). Preadipocytes were isolated from the tissue using a systematically modified enzymatic digestion procedure (Rodbell, 1964). The tissue was minced and incubated in digestion solution containing 1 mg Type I collagenase (Worthington Biochemical, Lakewood, NJ) and 1 mg bovine serum albumin (Sigma) per 1 mL Dulbecco's modified Eagle medium (DMEM) (Invitrogen, Carlsbad, CA) for 60 minutes at 37°C and 5% CO_2. The resulting suspension was filtered and centrifuged to isolate the cells. The cells were seeded in T-25 culture flasks with DMEM supplemented with 50 ml fetal bovine serum (Mediatech, Herndon, VA), 2 mL insulin-transferrin-sodium-selenite (Sigma), 1 mL fungizone (Invitrogen), and 5 mL antibiotic-antimycotic (Amphotericin B, penicillin, streptomycin; Invitrogen). At confluence, the cells were passaged to larger culture flasks, and then to roller bottles to obtain a sufficient number of cells from each animal that could be used for seeding onto beads.

5.2.3 Cell Seeding

Preliminary studies to identify optimal seeding conditions for each bead type were performed (results not shown here). It was determined that cells sufficiently attached to gelatin beads when cultured in stir flasks, while cells sufficiently attached to PL beads when cultured in roller bottles. The cells from each of the three heifers were cultured on both the gelatin and PL beads, with two stir flasks of gelatin beads and two roller bottles of PL beads prepared for each animal. The cells were cultured on the beads at an initial seeding density of 5×10^6 cells/mL beads for 7 days. Stir flasks were continuously stirred at 30 revolutions per minute using a multi-position stirrer (Barnstead-Thermolyne, Dubuque, IA), and roller bottles were continuously rotated at five revolutions per hour using a roller apparatus (Wheaton, Millville, NJ). All culture vessels were incubated at 37°C and 5% CO_2. A viability assay, a triglyceride assay, and reverse transcription polymerase chain reaction (RT-PCR) were used to evaluate cell viability, cellular activity, and characteristic gene expression, respectively.

5.2.4 Cell Viability Assessment

A LIVE/DEAD® Viability/Cytotoxicity Kit (Molecular Probes, Eugene, OR) was used to qualitatively assess cellular attachment to the gelatin and PL scaffolds and assess cellular viability after 7 days of culture on the beads and before the scaffolds were implanted into the heifers. The LIVE/DEAD® working solution was prepared in a sterile 15-mL centrifuge tube according to the manufacturer's instructions. Images of each sample were captured using the Axiovert 135 fluorescence inverted microscope (Zeiss, Thornwood, NY), a SPOT INSIGHT color digital camera (Diagnostic Instruments, Sterling Heights, MI), and Image Pro Plus 4.1 software (Media Cybernetics, Silver Spring, MD). Cellular bead samples of 200 μL, from each culture vessel, were evaluated for green and red fluorescence, indicative of viable and nonviable cells, respectively.

5.2.5 Triglyceride Measurement

The total triglyceride concentration within the cells was measured using a Cultured Human Adipocyte Differentiation Assay Kit (Zen-Bio, Inc., Research Triangle Park, NC). Under sterile conditions, a 200-μL sample of scaffolds was transferred from each of the 12 culture vessels to individual wells of a 12-well plate. The medium was aspirated from the scaffolds and 1 mL of sterile PBS was added to each well to rinse the scaffolds. The PBS was aspirated and 1 mL of a 0.5% solution of Triton-X-100 (Fisher Scientific, Middletown, VA) was added to each well to lyse the cells on the scaffolds. The scaffolds were then incubated at room temperature for 30 minutes. Following incubation, 20 μL of the sample lysate plus 80 μL of PBS were pipetted in triplicate, from each sample well, into three corresponding wells of a 96-well plate. Glycerol standards of concentrations ranging from 0 to 200 μM were prepared by diluting glycerol (Sigma) with an appropriate volume of sterile Millipore water from a Milli-Q Water System (Millipore, Bedford, MA). Next, 100 μL of Infinity™ triglyceride reagent (ThermoElectron Corporation, Melbourne, Australia) was added to each well of the plate containing either a standard or lysate sample. The plate was covered and incubated while protected from light for 15 minutes at room temperature. The absorbance of the samples in the plate was read at 490 nm using a spectrophotometer (MRX Revelation TC, Dynex Technologies, Chantilly, VA). A standard curve was prepared, plotting absorbance versus concentration of the prepared glycerol standard solutions. The average triglyceride concentration for all cell samples grown on a specific surface was reported.

5.2.6 Real-Time Polymerase Chain Reaction

Real-time polymerase chain reaction (RT-PCR) was used to determine if the cells cultured on the bead scaffolds expressed selected genes characteristic of preadipocytes or adipocytes. Samples from three different culture time points were evaluated: before culturing cells on beads (two-dimensional [2-D] culture), after 4 days of culture on bead scaffolds, and

TABLE 5.1   Primer Sequences for Target Genes

Target Gene	Sense Primer (5′→3′)	Antisense Primer (3′→5′)	Amplicon Size (bp)
β-actin	AGGCTCTCTTCCAGCCTTCC	TGTTGGCGTAGAGGTCCTTG	114
PPAR-γ	ACCACTCCCATGCCTTTGAC	AACCATCGGGTCAGCTCTTG	107
aP-2	GCTGCACTTCTTTCTCACCTTG	CCAGCCACTTTCCTGGTAGC	149
GADD 153	CCGTGGACAAGAACAGCAAC	TCACTGGTCAGCTCCAGCAC	130

after 7 days of culture on bead scaffolds. Primers, as shown in Table 5.1, specific for bovine growth arrest and deoxyribonucleic acid (DNA) damage inducible gene 153 (GADD 153), bovine peroxisome proliferator activator receptor-gamma (PPAR-γ), bovine adipocyte-specific fatty-acid-binding protein-2 (aP-2), and bovine beta-actin (β-actin), were designed for use in the RT-PCR analysis. GADD 153 was the gene selected to identify cells in the preadipocyte stage of differentiation. PPAR-γ and aP-2 were selected to identify cells in the mature adipocyte stage of differentiation; and β-actin was used as a housekeeping gene.

Total ribonucleic acid (RNA) was isolated from the samples using the reagents and instructions supplied in an RNeasy Mini Kit (QIAGEN, Valencia, CA). The concentration and purity of the isolated RNA samples was measured using an Agilent 2100 Bioanalyzer (Agilent Technologies, Inc., San Jose, CA). RT-PCR was performed using a OneStep RT-PCR Kit (QIAGEN), and RT-PCR reactions were conducted using a Mastercycler Gradient Thermal Cycler (Eppendorf, Hamburg, Germany). Gel electrophoresis was used to evaluate the RT-PCR products of the isolated cell sample reactions. A 2% agarose gel (Invitrogen) stained with ethidium bromide (0.5 µg/mL) (Bio-Rad, Hercules, CA) was prepared, and samples were loaded into the gel with a 100 basepair DNA ladder (Promega, Madison, WI). Electrophoresis was conducted for 2 hours at 5 kV/cm (Model FB300, Fisher Scientific). The gel was then viewed using a UV-Spectroline® BI-O-Vision™ UV/White Light Transilluminator (Spectronics Corporation, Westbury, NY) and a GEL LOGIC 100 Imaging System equipped with 1D Image Analysis Software (Kodak, Rochester, NY).

5.2.7 Implant Sample Preparation

The implant samples were loaded into 3-cc syringes (Tyco Healthcare, Mansfield, MA) fitted with 14-gauge needles (Sherwood Medical, St. Louis, MO) under sterile conditions in a laminar flow hood in the laboratory and then were transported to the dairy farm for implantation. Syringes containing a calcium chloride gelling solution, alginate carrier, saline solution, and acellular bead samples were prepared first, and those containing cellular bead samples were prepared last. All syringes were stored in a warming travel carrier and were maintained at 37°C (Vector, Ft. Lauderdale, FL) until injection. Six total implant combinations, consisting of four experimental samples with both cellular and acellular bead scaffolds, and two control samples, were prepared (72 total sample syringes). Specifically, the implants comprised:

- Alginate carrier + cellular PL beads

- Alginate carrier + cellular gelatin beads

- Alginate carrier + acellular PL beads

- Alginate carrier + acellular gelatin beads

- Alginate carrier

- Saline

The total volume for each implanted sample was 1.25 mL. The total volume of the saline control sample consisted solely of sterile 0.9% sodium chloride (Baxter Healthcare, Corp., Deerfield, IL). The alginate carrier sample consisted of 1 mL of 1% w/v alginate solution prepared by dissolving 1 g of alginic acid (Acros Organics, Geel, Belgium) in distilled water; that solution was then mixed with 0.25 mL of sterile 0.05 M calcium chloride solution (Fisher Chemicals, Fair Lawn, NJ) to gel the alginate at the time of injection. Each of the samples containing beads consisted of 0.5 mL of the specified bead type, 0.5 mL of 1% w/v alginate solution, and 0.25 mL 0.05 M calcium chloride. The calcium chloride was loaded into separate 3-cc syringes; sterile Argyle® EZ-Flo three-way stopcocks (Sherwood Medical) were used to allow mixing of the alginate or the alginate-containing beads immediately before injection into the animals.

5.2.8 Implantation and Retrieval

Following intravenous (i.v.) administration of acepromazine (Vedco), a 3-row × 4-column rectangular grid pattern was shaved onto the left and right sides of each of the three heifers (Figure 5.1a). Implants were injected intradermally at the lower left corner of each square. The animals were held in a recovery pen for 2 days post injection, after which time they were relocated to a holding pen until the biopsy of the samples was performed. The implanted samples on the left side of each heifer were biopsied 11 days post implantation, while the samples on the right side were biopsied 27 days post implantation (Figure 5.1c and d). For implant biopsies, the heifers were sedated with i.v. administration of acepromazine. After cleaning the injection sites with Betadine® solution (Purdue Frederick Co.), lidocaine (Vedco) was injected locally at each site to be biopsied, a scalpel incision was made at the lower left corner of the shaved areas, and the tissue containing the implant sample was excised from the animal. The site of tissue removal was then sutured using absorbable sutures (Figure 5.1b), and the side of the animal was sprayed with Betadine® (Purdue Frederick Co.) and Catron IV fly spray (Bayer Healthcare LLC, Shawnee Mission, KS). Biozide® wound gel (Performance Products, Inc.) was also applied to the sutured sites. Antibiotics, i.v. Banamine® (Schering-Plough Animal Health, Kenilworth, NJ) and intramuscular Excenel® (Pfizer Animal Health, Florham Park, NJ), were administered to each animal immediately post operation and again 2 days postoperatively, during which time the animals were held in a recovery pen. The animals were returned to normal housing following the postoperative period after the final time point.

5.2.9 Histological Processing and Assessment

Tissue samples were fixed in 10% neutral buffered formalin (Fisher Chemicals, Fair Lawn, NJ). Paraffin-embedded samples were sectioned, and the resulting tissue sections were stained

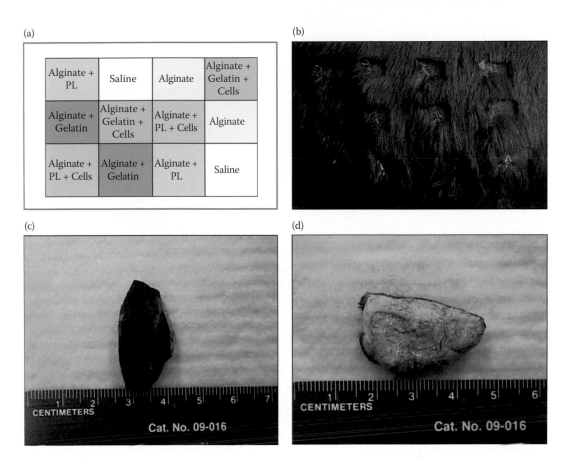

(a)

Alginate + PL	Saline	Alginate	Alginate + Gelatin + Cells
Alginate + Gelatin	Alginate + Gelatin + Cells	Alginate + PL + Cells	Alginate
Alginate + PL + Cells	Alginate + Gelatin	Alginate + PL	Saline

(b)

(c)

CENTIMETERS

Cat. No. 09-016

(d)

CENTIMETERS

Cat. No. 09-016

FIGURE 5.1 The implant samples were injected on the left and right sides of each heifer according to the specified grid pattern (a), with injections targeted for the lower left corner of each shaved square. The implanted samples were biopsied and then were sutured, with sutured sites appearing as shown 4 days following the biopsy procedure (b). Representative images of the skin side (c) and underside (d) of the biopsied tissue samples.

with hematoxylin and eosin (H&E) (Richard-Allan Scientific, Kalamazoo, MI) and Masson's Trichrome (Poly Scientific, Bay Shore, NY). Two H&E-stained sections of each sample were used for the histological assessment. Images, at increasing objective magnifications of 4–40×, of a representative area of the implant on each of the histology slides were captured using a Nikon Eclipse E600 microscope (Nikon Corporation Nikon Instech Co., Ltd., Tokyo, Japan) with a QImaging MicroPublisher 3.3 camera (QImaging Corporation, Surrey, BC, Canada) using QCapture 2.70.0 software (QImaging Corporation, Surrey, BC, Canada). The identity of each captured image was hidden; subsequently, each image was independently reviewed by two investigators and qualitatively assessed using an adapted semiquantitative rating system to assess capsule formation at the interface of the implant material, inflammatory response based on the presence of inflammatory cells within the samples, tissue ingrowth within the implant material, and development of new adipose tissue (Jansen *et al.*, 1994). The specific criterion used by investigators to evaluate each sample is detailed in Table 5.2. A score of 0, 1, 2, 3, or 4 was assigned by the investigators

TABLE 5.2   Criteria for Histological Assessment

Capsule Formation at Implant Interface		Inflammatory Reaction	
Evaluate the quality of the option zone tissue immediately surrounding the implant		Evaluate the inflammatory response of the host to the implanted samples relative to the provided representative images of inflammation levels	
Response	**Score**	**Response**	**Score**
Reactive tissue is fibrous, mature, not dense, resembling connective or fat tissue in the noninjured regions	4	Tissue resembles the normal tissue section and there are little to no inflammatory cells present in the sample. (Fibroblasts contact implant surface without presence of macrophages or foreign body giant cells)	4
Reactive tissue is fibrous but immature, showing fibroblasts and little collagen	3	Few inflammatory cells present in the section but there is the presence of some. (Scattered macrophages and foreign body giant cells present)	3
Reactive tissue is granulous and dense, containing both fibroblasts and many inflammatory cells	2	Inflammatory cells present but not excessive. (One layer of macrophages and foreign body giant cells present)	2
Reactive tissue consists of masses of inflammatory cells with little or no signs of connective tissue organization	1	Tissue resembles the representative "high" level of inflammation for the sample set. Level of inflammation appears excessive/extreme (Multiple layers of macrophages and foreign body giant cells present	1
Cannot be evaluated because of infection or other factors not necessarily related to the material	0	Cannot be evaluated because of infection or other factors not necessarily related to the material	0
Interstitial Tissue Assessment		**New Adipose Tissue Development**	
Evaluate the presence or lack of new vasculature formed within the interstitial space of implanted samples		Evaluate the presence or lack of new adipose tissue formation within the implanted samples	
Response	**Score**	**Response**	**Score**
Tissue in interstitium shows blood vessels, is fibrous, mature, not dense, resembling connective or fat tissue in the normal tissue section	4	Adipose tissue is visibly present within the sample	4
Tissue in interstitium shows young fibroblasts invading the spaces, not macrophages present, but connective tissue is evident	3		3
Tissue in interstitium shows giant cells and other inflammatory cells in abundance but connective components in between	2		2
Tissue in interstitium is dense and exclusively of the inflammatory type	1	No adipose tissue visibly present within the sample	1
Cannot be evaluated because of infection or other factors not necessarily related to the material	0	Cannot be evaluated because of infection or other factors not necessarily related to the material	0

to assess the images, with a score of 0 assigned for a minimal response and a score of 4 assigned for a maximum response.

5.2.10 Statistical Analyses

Paired *t*-tests were used with a significance level of $\alpha=0.05$ to make comparisons for triglyceride analysis. The experimental design used for the implantation study was a randomized block design. Blocks were assigned based on the individual heifers, and the treatments were based on the specific implant types for each time point (12 treatments). All statistical analyses were performed using SAS 9.1 (SAS Institute Inc., Cary, NC). The least squares mean was used with a significance level of $\alpha=0.05$ to determine significant differences.

5.3 RESULTS

Representative images of the cells at each stage are shown to demonstrate the progression of the growth of the cells *in vitro*. Immediately following the isolation procedure, the cells in the culture flasks appeared rounded in shape, small in diameter, and were not attached to the surface of the flasks (Figure 5.2a). By Day 10 of culture, the cells were noticeably proliferating. The cells were attached to the culture flask and were fusiform in shape, which is characteristic of preadipocytes (Figure 5.2b). On Day 14, the cells had increased in number. At this point, they also appeared more rounded in shape, and were accumulating lipid as is characteristic of differentiating adipocytes (Figure 5.2c). On viewing the cells at higher magnification, lipid droplets were visible within the cells (Figure 5.2d).

5.3.1 Cell Viability Assessment

Images of the cells stained for LIVE/DEAD analysis after 7 days of culture showed a large number of viable cells attached to the gelatin beads for all heifers. Representative images (Figure 5.3a and b) show cells cultured on the gelatin microcarriers and completely covering the individual beads. A low number of dead cells were visible on the gelatin beads at this time point for each of the cultures. On Day 7 of PL bead cultures, cellular attachment was not as consistent. The cells seemed to attach readily to some PL beads for each of the heifers, as evidenced by individual beads covered with viable cells. There were, however, several PL beads in the culture vessels for each heifer that had little to no cells attached (Figure 5.3b and 5.3c).

5.3.2 Triglyceride Measurement

To further characterize the cells cultured on the injectable beads, an assay measuring the total triglyceride concentration of the cells was conducted. The cells were initially cultured on 2-D surfaces of tissue culture-treated polystyrene flasks. Prior to seeding onto the beads, the cells produced a minimal amount of triglyceride (Figure 5.4a). However, following culture of the cells on the beads for 4 days, the triglyceride concentration increased for cells seeded on both the gelatin and PL bead types, with a significant increase measured for the cells cultured on the PL beads ($p < 0.05$). The cells seeded on the gelatin microcarriers also exhibited a significant increase in triglyceride concentration on Day 7; but by Day 7, a

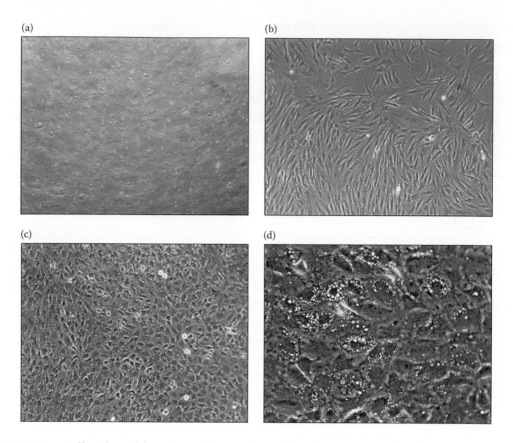

FIGURE 5.2   Cells cultured for 1 day in tissue culture flasks (a) were rounded and were not attached to the surface. By Day 10, the cell number increased (b), and the fusiform morphology of the cells was evident. Cells cultured for 14 days in flasks became rounded (c) and, on viewing at higher magnification (d), lipid droplets were visible within the cells. Photographs a, b, and c were taken at 100× total magnification; Photograph d was taken at 320× total magnification.

significant decrease in the triglyceride content, compared with Day 4 values, was observed in the PL cultures.

5.3.3 RT-PCR

The RT-PCR products of RNA samples isolated from cells seeded on beads were evaluated using gel electrophoresis. The resulting gel electrophoresis images showed that the cells cultured on the 2-D surfaces before seeding onto beads (designated Day 0) only actively expressed β-actin and did not express any of the adipogenic genes (Figure 5.4b). After 4 days of culture on the gelatin microcarriers, β-actin expression was detected in two of the three tested samples, along with faint expression of aP-2 and PPAR-γ in those same samples (Figure 5.4c). After 4 days of culture on the PL scaffolds, the β-actin gene was detected in two of the three samples; however, none of the adipogenic genes was detected (Figure 5.4d). Following 7 days of culture on the gelatin scaffolds, β-actin was expressed by all cell samples; however, no adipogenic genes were expressed (Figure 5.4c). Similar findings were observed for cells cultured on PL beads for 7 days (Figure 5.4d).

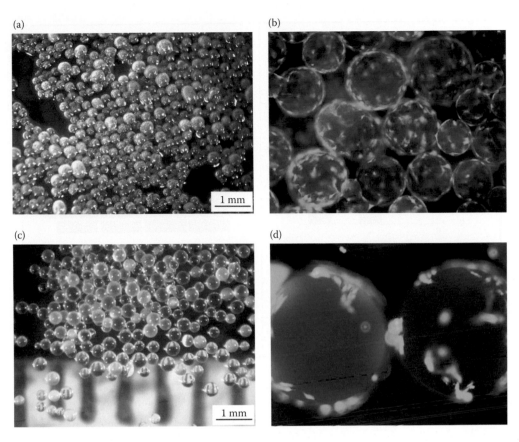

FIGURE 5.3 Representative stereomicroscope images of gelatin microcarriers (a) and PL beads (c) following hydration and fabrication, respectively. Live/Dead images showing cells seeded on gelatin microcarriers (b) and on PL beads (d) following 7 days of culture, using a 10× objective.

5.3.4 Histological Assessment

Evaluation of histological scores assigned to the saline controls biopsied from the heifers showed that the scores for each category remained constant throughout the experiment, with no significant change in any category, between Day 11 and Day 27 for the control samples. Representative images of the control tissue stained with H&E and Masson's Trichrome, as shown in Figure 5.5a and b, respectively, demonstrate the appearance of normal tissue that all other experimental samples were compared to for assessment and scoring. Comparison of the scores for each sample containing implant material (alginate alone, or alginate with cellular and acellular beads gelatin, Figure 5.5c–f, or PL) to the saline control showed that the scores for each implant type were significantly different in each category of assessment, with the exception of the formation of new adipose tissue.

The results of assessment of the implant interface, the reactive zone immediately surrounding the implants, are shown in Figure 5.5g. Histological analysis of the samples indicates a general decline in the assigned score of the tissue at the implant interface from Day 11 to Day 27 for the acellular and cellular implants of both gelatin and PL bead types. In most cases, the reactive zone tissue appeared fibrous, but not completely mature as found

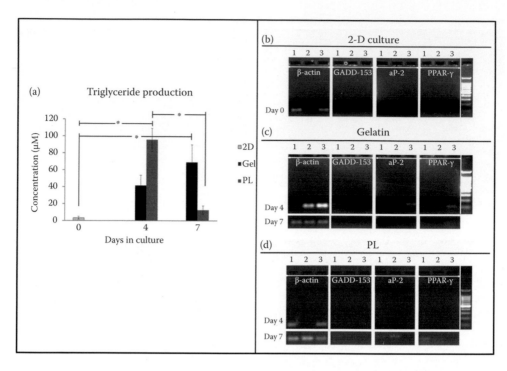

FIGURE 5.4 (a) Concentrations of triglyceride measured in cells cultured in 2-D and on the gelatin and PL bead specified time points. Increased triglyceride concentrations were measured in cells cultured on 3-D surfaces as compared with 2-D culture. Error bars represent standard error of the mean (SEM). Asterisks (∗) indicate significant statistical difference ($p < 0.05$). Gel electrophoresis results for cell samples cultured on 2-D surfaces did not express any adipogenic markers on Day 0 (b). When cultured on gelatin microcarriers (c) and PL beads (d) for 4 days, expression of adipogenic markers was only observed in cells cultured on gelatin microcarriers. On Day 7, there was not any expression of adipogenic markers observed in cells cultured on gelatin microcarriers (c) or PL beads (d).

in the control tissue. The addition of cells to the gelatin and PL beads had little effect on the implant interface scores. Each sample type consistently included a thin capsule surrounding the implant material (Figure 5.5e and f). Additionally, there was no statistically significant difference in histology scores for the implant interface when samples of acellular or cellular beads types from Day 11 to Day 27 were compared (Figure 5.5g).

The inflammatory responses elicited by the implant samples were also qualitatively assessed with scores assigned as shown in Figure 5.5h. When compared to the control tissue samples, each of the implant types elicited some form of inflammatory response. The largest response was found in the cellular and acellular samples containing gelatin beads. Over time, from Day 11 to Day 27, the level of inflammation for the samples containing gelatin and PL beads tended to increase, although the increase was not statistically significant. When cells were added to the gelatin and PL beads, there was no statistically significant effect on the level of inflammation of the samples when compared to the corresponding acellular samples of each bead type. The acellular and cellular gelatin beads, however, tended to elicit a higher inflammatory reaction, although not statistically significant, than the corresponding

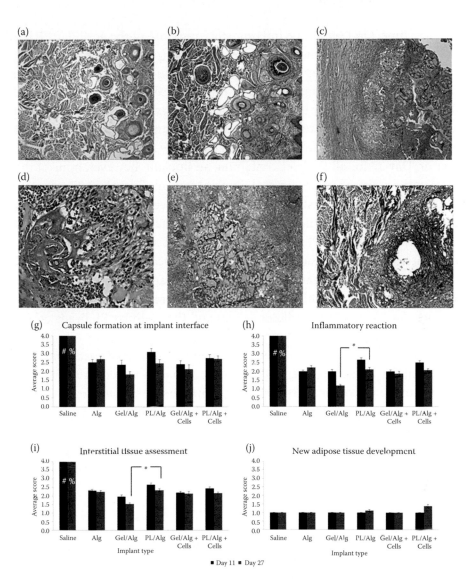

FIGURE 5.5   Unless noted, all magnifications of 4× objective. Representative hematoxylin & eosin (H&E) (a) and Masson's Trichrome stained sections (b), respectively, of the normal bovine control skin tissue samples, which received saline injections. Following 27 days of implantation, gelatin (c) and PL (not shown here) beads were still apparent within the tissue samples as evidenced by the clearly rounded structures within the sample. At higher magnification, 20× objective magnification, degradation of the gelatin beads is portrayed by the scalloped bead edges (d). A thin capsule consistently formed, surrounding the implant material, shown here in a gelatin sample stained with H&E (e) and Masson's Trichrome (f). Scores assigned for semiquantitative assessment of the capsule formed at the interface of the implanted samples (g), the inflammatory reaction of the tissue to the implanted samples (h), and the quality of the interstitial tissue within the implant samples (i) indicate a general decline in scores for all samples containing implants when compared to the control tissue. No new adipose tissue was observed within any samples (j). Error bars represent SEM. Asterisks (∗) indicate significant statistical difference ($p < 0.05$). The pound sign (#) and percent sign (%) indicate values statistically different from all other values ($p < 0.05$).

PL groups over time. On Day 27, the inflammatory response of the acellular PL beads was significantly lower than that of the acellular gelatin beads ($p < 0.05$) (Figure 5.5h).

Scores assigned to the samples when evaluated for tissue ingrowth within the interstitium of the implant are shown in Figure 5.5i. The presence of new vasculature within the implant was not observed in any of the histological samples. The scores for tissue ingrowth for samples containing an implant were generally less than the score assigned to the control tissue samples. Over time, from Day 11 to Day 27, the interstitial tissue scores tended to be lower on Day 27 for all samples containing an implant; however, none of the differences between the assigned values for each implant type on Day 11 or 27 was statistically significant on comparison. Interstitial tissue scores of the cellular and acellular PL samples also tended to be higher than the scores of samples containing gelatin beads. The addition of cells to the gelatin and PL beads again had no statistically significant effect on the interstitial scores assigned for each sample. Of the two bead types, the interstitial scores of samples containing gelatin beads tended to be lower than those of acellular and cellular PL beads. However, the only statistically significant difference observed was between the assigned scores for tissue of the acellular gelatin and the acellular PL beads on Day 27 of the study ($p < 0.05$) (Figure 5.5i).

The samples were assessed to determine if new adipose tissue developed from the implantation of the cellular tissue-engineered constructs, with data as shown in Figure 5.5j. No visible adipose tissue was observed in any of the control tissue samples. Furthermore, there was no visible adipose tissue observed in any of samples containing bead material. The adipose tissue observed in the acellular PL/alginate and the cellular PL/alginate biopsies on Day 27 was presumed to be subcutaneous fat already present in the sample. No new adipose tissue formation was observed in any of the samples receiving an injection consisting of cellular beads (Figure 5.5j).

5.4 DISCUSSION

The overall goal of this research was to construct and evaluate tissue engineered injectable devices for breast tissue reconstruction, while demonstrating the utility of a relevant large animal model, specific to human breast tissue engineering. A quick review of the literature reveals thousands of breast cancer studies involving rats or mice; however, there are only approximately 40 studies involving breast cancer and cows. The former include hundreds of tissue engineering studies; the latter include none. Certainly, the selection of a rodent model is driven by finances, by animal housing constraints, by historical precedence and the need for data comparability between studies, and by availability of relevant assays and techniques (e.g., immunohistochemistry). However, the amount of information that one can glean from a model that is dissimilar to human in size, biochemistry, and physicomechanics is limited; it is, therefore, time that we look to incorporate relevant large animal models. Cows and sheep are much larger in mass than rodents; the effect of the implant material on the overall biological environment in a cow or sheep is significantly less than it would be in a rodent, where the implant/host ratio is larger. This point is not trivial when considering absorbable systems that rely on efficient transport to remove acidic by-products. The implant/host ratio in cows and sheep is far more similar to that in humans than the implant/host ratio in rodents. It is also important to remember that different large animal species can provide a wide range of options to allow assessment of a wide range of biomedical questions. For example, the gestation periods for relevant large animal models vary; the gestation periods for cows (280–284 days) are much closer to humans (266 days) than for sheep (~148 days).

The bovine model that we pursued provides important animal welfare considerations with respect to the 3Rs – refinement, reduction, and replacement. Addressing refinement, we used Generally Regarded as Safe (GRAS) materials that are safe for human ingestion and, accordingly, we were able to reduce the animal number by avoiding the need for euthanasia. Additionally, we used an intradermal surgical site to achieve a minimally invasive surgery. The intradermal location was possible due to the thickness of cow skin and would not be possible in a rodent, which has very thin skin. Regarding reduction, because the cow is a large animal with high surface area, we were able to assess multiple implants on one animal. A rodent model would necessitate multiple animals to support the same breadth of data. Also, the intradermal site allows the samples to be contained and readily captured, so we were able to minimize variability and animal number (we would need a larger number of rodents to accommodate the dispersion of samples at the implant site and subsequent difficulties in identification and retrieval). And regarding replacement, use of an inbred rat model, for example, would necessitate inclusion of donor rats in the study; by having an animal large enough to allow autologous implants, we were able to reduce the number of animals in the study. Also, we conducted a significant amount of *in vitro* work in an attempt to refine the cellular systems; so, significantly less developmental work was needed *in vivo*.

Isolated cells from the heifers exhibited morphology characteristic of mature adipocytes, as shown by representative images of cells in 2-D culture before seeding onto the beads. However, the lack of adipogenic markers expressed by cells cultured in 2-D, as shown by gel electrophoresis results, and the negligible amount of lipid measured by triglyceride assay suggests that these cells may have undergone dedifferentiation with passage and doubling in 2-D culture (Ailhaud, 1982; Cawthorn *et al.*, 2012; Fernyhough *et al.*, 2005a, b; Vierck *et al.*, 2001). The increase in triglyceride concentration following culture on both the gelatin and PL 3-D scaffolds demonstrates one advantage of 3-D cultures, whereby cells may undergo differentiation without the need for adipogenic stimuli. The 3-D cultures provide greater culture surface for cells that contributes to an increase in cell number as cells proliferate over that increased area. The culture of cells on 3-D beads also likely encourages increased cell-cell contact that lead to further cell differentiation and the increased lipid production observed by triglyceride assay when 3-D gelatin and PL samples are compared to the 2-D samples.

While culture on both the gelatin and PL 3-D scaffolds resulted in greater triglyceride production and in the expression of some adipogenic markers than what was observed in 2-D samples, there was a difference in the response of cells to the different materials. The amount of triglyceride measured in cells on gelatin beads increased from Day 4 to Day 7 in culture, while cells on PL beads exhibited a significant decrease in triglyceride over time. Cells cultured on gelatin beads also exhibited some expression of aP-2 and PPAR-γ;

however, no expression of adipogenic markers was detected by cells on PL beads at any point of culturing. With the greatest amount of triglyceride measured in the samples cultured on PL beads for 4 days, one would have expected to observe expression of adipogenic markers with RT-PCR. It is important to note that adipogenic markers may have been expressed, but due to low RNA concentration, the level may have been too low for detection at our amplification conditions. The decrease in triglyceride noted in the PL samples, however, is likely due to a loss of cells that were securely attached to the scaffolds by Day 7. The loss of cells from the PL beads means there would be fewer cells proliferating, which would result in slowed differentiation, as indicated by the lack of adipogenic markers on Day 7 for PL samples.

The gelatin beads, however, seemed to continually support the proliferation and differentiation of cells such that they produced increasing levels of triglyceride and expressed adipogenic markers, indicating the presence of mature adipocytes. The cells on gelatin beads, however, did not express adipogenic markers on Day 7 of culture, which may have resulted from low RNA concentration. As cell behavior is proven to be influenced by many aspects of a biomaterial's surface, including surface chemistry and topography (Alves *et al.*, 2010; Bacakova *et al.*, 2007; Boyan *et al.*, 1996; García, 2006), these differences in cellular response to each surface may be attributed to the differences that exist between the gelatin and PL materials. As a synthetic biomaterial, PL has been widely used for tissue engineering applications; however, because of its hydrophobic nature, PL has low affinity for cell attachment because of its lack of cell binding sites. Polymer modification methods are often used to improve cell-biomaterial interactions for PL (Třesohlavá *et al.*, 2009; Wang *et al.*, 2005), such as the method of hydrolysis (soaking in ethanol) that was used for the PL beads fabricated for this study. Gelatin is a natural biomaterial derived from denatured collagen and is recognized by cells, leading to high cell affinity to the material (Gomillion and Burg, 2011). While cells initially attached to the PL beads, the level of attachment was visibly less than on the gelatin beads, as shown by Live/Dead images. In addition, previous characterization of the surface topography of the gelatin and PL beads with scanning electron microscopy showed the gelatin beads to be highly porous and textured, while the PL beads were relatively smooth (Cavin, 2005; Gomillion *et al.*, 2007). While initially attached to both bead types, the differences in surface chemistry and texture may have also contributed to easy shearing of cells from the PL surface while in roller bottle culture, leading to fewer cells available on PL beads to differentiate and produce triglyceride during the culture period. These properties of the gelatin and PL beads also assuredly affected cellular attachment during preparation of the implant samples and subsequent injection into the heifers.

The implantation of the composite devices containing PL beads was not completely successful due to bead aggregation in the syringes that caused the needles to become clogged in some instances. The histological samples containing PL scaffolds, therefore, tended to more closely resemble the control tissue samples, which represented tissue response due to saline injection. Hence, a direct histological comparison between PL and gelatin-based composite systems must consider the substantially lower number of cellular PL beads implanted. However, one would expect to tune each composite to the appropriate ratio of cells to biomaterial and one would not expect this ratio to be equivalent from biomaterial type to type. In fact, one would want to consider the characteristics of the specific bio-material in order to optimize this ratio – for example, PL degrades into acidic products, naturally derived materials tend to elicit sharper, less tunable foreign body responses, and PL has no receptor sites to encourage cellular attachment, etc.

The increase in the level of inflammation during the implantation period for each implanted material is likely due to a chronic response to the sample injections and presence of foreign material. It was expected that the gelatin microcarriers would be remod-eled relatively quickly since they are derived from a natural material, but this was not the case. The slow degradation can be largely attributed to the degree of cross-linking of the microcarriers. The gelatin microcarriers, according to manufacturer's specifications, were cross-linked with hexamethylene diisocyanate, which provides high thermal and mechanical stability. Interestingly, the presence of a large number of cells, which would generally work to remodel the gelatin, did not have such an effect on these microcarriers during this implantation period because of their increased mechanical stability.

The overall goal of this work was to induce the formation of new adipose tissue *in vivo* with the implantation of these minimally invasive injectable devices. The lack of newly developed adipose tissue and/or adipocytes may be attributed to the de-differentiation of the implanted adipose cells and the lack of optimization of the composite system. The cells at the time of implantation were fibroblast-like in a de-differentiated state and, therefore, did not have the capability for differentiating or inducing new fat tissue production without an added stimulus. It is possible in primary culture for a small number of contaminating fibroblasts to rapidly overtake a culture population. Fibroblasts would be impossible to visually differentiate from preadipocytes in primary culture; hence, in future work, the cultures should be further characterized to determine fibroblast presence. One could argue that the culture should be purified; however, it may be that a heterogeneous population of cells, similar to that found in native tissue, allows the appropriate signals between cells types. Following this line of thought, one would still want to characterize and then opti-mize the cellular distribution. In addition, several preliminary tests were conducted, prior to the execution of this bovine study, to identify the best logistical methods for handling sample injections. Live/Dead analysis also indicated high cellular content on bead samples; however, future work should certainly address the shearing effect on cell attachment to the bead surfaces as well as the optimal cell concentration for implants and the level of cell maturity post injection. For example, the number of cells implanted with each sam-ple in the bovine study may simply not have been large enough to induce new adipose tissue formation *in vivo*. It has been shown that adipose tissue development results from the growth of adipocyte cells in size and the increase in adipocyte cell number, such that the recruitment of new fat cells *in vivo* is dependent on the proliferation and differentiation of preadipocytes in fat deposits (Peixing *et al.*, 2001). If, in the implanted samples, there was not a viable population of actively differentiating and proliferating preadipocytes on the beads, then there would be no stimulus, or the present cells may not have the capacity for adipose tissue formation within the intradermal space of the heifers, just as we had observed.

The presence of cellular components surrounding individual beads of the implanted samples suggests the feasibility of the injectable composite to allow tissue infiltration within the injectable composite; however, the lack of new adipose tissue formation within the implanted samples indicates that further modification of the implant may be necessary. Future studies should begin with verification of the adipogenic potential of the isolated cells from the adipose tissue samples. Other factors related to the use of primary adipose cells should also be considered. The basis for the proposed devices stems from the idea of using an injectable composite device for restoring tissue. The idea of using a composite may be expanded to form implants consisting of different beads that will serve specific purposes. For example, the PL beads used for forming implants supported less cell attachment than the gelatin microcarriers, and the cells were shown to easily detach from the surface of the beads. The PL beads may be better suited for a different purpose in the composite system – simply as slow-degrading materials that help maintain mechanical integrity or as slow-releasing vehicles for local administration of growth factors or other cell stimuli that could enhance the adipogenic differentiation capacity of implanted cells or recruit cells to the implant site. PL scaffolds have been investigated, for example, as drug delivery agents where substances may be encapsulated into the microcarriers, and other materials, such as chitosan, have been evaluated in our laboratory for such purposes in the injectable composite system. Growth factors and differentiation-inducing stimuli could potentially be incorporated into the device, resulting in a highly tunable system that could be tailored to specific patient needs and that could be used to enhance the overall implant efficacy for tissue reconstruction.

5.5 CONCLUSION

The overall goals of this work were to evaluate the feasibility of using a bovine model for assessing tissue-engineered injectable devices for breast tissue reconstruction and demonstrate the ability of the composite to allow tissue infiltration. We successfully showed the use of a bovine model that could be implemented for clinically relevant evaluation of biomaterial-based systems and the significant advantages afforded by this large animal model, particularly with respect to animal welfare considerations of the 3Rs (refinement, reduction, and replacement). With this initial proof-of-concept study, the foundation has been laid for further development of this large animal model system. Based on the qualitative and quantitative histological analyses, the overall goal of inducing adipose tissue formation *in vivo* was not accomplished with this study; however, the cellular materials can readily be optimized to improve this outcome. It was shown, however, that unlike traditional bulk scaffolds, cellular injectable tissue-engineered devices that incorporated gelatin and PL beads, indeed, allow cellular infiltration throughout the entire implant volume post implantation, which is a crucial finding on which optimization studies can now be built. Further assessment of cell isolation and culturing techniques are required to address the issues of long-term tissue bulking and maintenance, which is critical for improving the system's efficacy for breast reconstruction. This research is the first reported use of a bovine model for a tissue engineering system; the results demonstrate the tremendous potential of an alternative large animal model for preclinical testing of regenerative therapies.

ACKNOWLEDGMENTS

We gratefully acknowledge the staff at the Lamaster Dairy Center for their assistance. This study was supported, in part, by the National Science Foundation Presidential Early Career Award for Scientists and Engineers (award #BES 0093805).

REFERENCES

Ailhaud G. 1982, Adipose cell differentiation in culture. *Mol Cell Biochem*, 49:17–31.

Ailhaud G, Grimaldi P, Negrel R. 1992, Cellular and molecular aspects of adipose tissue development. *Annu Rev Nutr*, 12:207–233.

Akers RM. 2002, *Lactation and the Mammary Gland*, Iowa State University Press, Ames, IA.

Alhadlaq A, Tang M, Mao JJ. 2005, Engineered adipose tissue from human mesenchymal stem cells maintains predefined shape and dimension: implications in soft tissue augmentation and reconstruction. *Tissue Eng*, 11:556–566.

Alluwaimi AM. 2004, The cytokines of bovine mammary gland: prospects for diagnosis and therapy, *Res Vet Sci*, 77:211–222.

Alves NM, Pashkuleva I, Reis RL, Mano JF. 2010, Controlling cell behavior through the design of polymer surfaces. *Small*, 6:2208–2220.

Atala A, Lanza RP. 2002, *Methods of Tissue Engineering*, Academic Press, San Diego, CA.

Bacakova L, Filova E, Kubies D, Machova L, Proks V, Malinova V, Lisa V, Rypacek F. 2007, Adhesion and growth of vascular smooth muscle cells in cultures on bioactive RGD peptide-carrying polylactides. *J Mater Sci: Mater Med*, 18:1317–1323.

Band MR, Larson JH, Rebeiz M, Green CA, Heyen DW, Donovan J, Windish R, Steining C, Mahyuddin P, Womack JE, Lewin HA. 2000, An ordered comparative map of the cattle and human genomes. *Genome Res*, 10:1359–1368.

Beahm EK, Walton RL, Patrick CW, Jr. 2003, Progress in adipose tissue construct development. *Clin Plast Surg*, 30:547–558.

Bierła JB, Osińska TM, Motyl T. 2012, Bovine mammary stem cells studies—current status—a review. *Anim Sci Pap Rep*, 30:195–204.

Borena BM, Bussche L, Burvenich C, Duchateau L, Van de Walle GR. 2013, Mammary stem cell research in veterinary science: an update. *Stem Cells Dev*, 22:1743–1751.

Boyan BD, Hummert TW, Dean DD, Schwartz Z. 1996, Role of material surfaces in regulating bone and cartilage cell response. *Biomaterials*, 17:137–146.

Brown RQ, Mount A, Burg KJ. 2005, Evaluation of polymer scaffolds to be used in a composite injectable system for intervertebral disc tissue engineering. *J Biomed Mater Res A*, 74:32–39.

Burg KJL, Austin CE, Culberson CR, Greene KG, Halberstadt CR, Holder WD, Jr., Loebsack AB, Roland WD. 2000, 'A novel approach to tissue engineering: injectable composites', in *Transactions of the 2000 World Biomaterials Congress*, Kamuela, HI.

Burg KJ, Boland T. 2003, Minimally invasive tissue engineering composites and cell printing. *IEEE EMB*, 22:84–91.

Burg KJL, Shalaby SW. 1999, 'Biodegradable materials,' in *Tissue Engineering of Prosthetic Vascular Grafts*, eds. Zilla P, Greisler HP, R.G. Landes Co., Austin, TX.

Capuco AV, Ellis S. 2005, Bovine mammary progenitor cells: current concepts and future directions. *J Mammary Gland Biol Neoplasia*, 10:5–15.

Cavin AN, Ellis SE, Burg KJL. 2005. Adipocyte Response to Injectable Breast Tissue Engineering Scaffolds. *Transactions of the 30th Annual Meeting of the Society For Biomaterials*, Memphis, TN.

Cawthorn WP, Scheller EL, MacDougald OA. 2012, Adipose tissue stem cells meet preadipocyte commitment: going back to the future. *J Lipid Res*, 53:227–246.

Chen G, Ushida T, Tateishi T. 2002, Scaffold design for tissue engineering. *Macromol Biosci*, 2:67–77.

Choi JH, Gimble JM, Lee K, Marra KG, Rubin JP, Yoo JJ, Vunjak-Novakovic G, Kaplan DL. 2010, Adipose tissue engineering for soft tissue regeneration. *Tissue Eng Part B Rev*, 16:413–426.

Choi YS, Park SN, Suh H. 2005, Adipose tissue engineering using mesenchymal stem cells attached to injectable PLGA spheres. *Biomaterials*, 26:5855–5863.

De Ugarte DA, Ashjian PH, Elbarbary A, Hedrick MH. 2003, Future of fat as raw material for tissue regeneration. *Ann Plast Surg*, 50:215–219.

Fernyhough ME, Bucci LR, Hausman GJ, Antonio J, Vierck JL, Dodson MV. 2005a, Gaining a solid grip on adipogenesis. *Tissue Cell*, 37:335–338.

Fernyhough ME, Helterline DL, Vierck JL, Hausman GJ, Hill RA, Dodson MV. 2005b, Dedifferentiation of mature adipocytes to form adipofibroblasts: more than just a possibility. *Adipocytes*, 1:17–24.

Ford TS, Ross MW, Acland HM, Madison JB. 1989, Primary teat neoplasia in two yearling heifers. *J Am Vet Med Assoc*, 195:238–239.

Fuchs JR, Nasseri BA, Vacanti JP. 2001, Tissue engineering: a 21st century solution to surgical reconstruction. *Ann Thorac Surg*, 72:577–591.

García A. 2006, 'Interfaces to control cell-biomaterial adhesive interactions', in *Polymers for Regenerative Medicine*, ed. Werner C, Springer, Berlin, Germany and Heidelberg, Germany, 171–190.

Gomillion CT, Burg KJ. 2006, Stem cells and adipose tissue engineering. *Biomaterials*, 27:6052–6063.

Gomillion CT, Burg KJL. 2011, 'Adipose tissue engineering,' in *Comprehensive Biomaterials*, ed. Paul D, Elsevier, Oxford, 529–539.

Gomillion CT, Parzel CA, White RL, Burg KJL. 2007, 'Tissue engineering: breast,' in *Encyclopedia of Biomaterials and Biomedical Engineering*, eds. Wnek GE, Bowlin GL, CRC Press, New York, 1–8.

Halberstadt C, Austin C, Rowley J, Culberson C, Loebsack A, Wyatt S, Coleman S, Blacksten L, Burg K, Mooney D, Holder W, Jr. 2002, A hydrogel material for plastic and reconstructive applications injected into the subcutaneous space of a sheep. *Tissue Eng*, 8:309–319.

Hemmrich K, von Heimburg D, Rendchen R, Di Bartolo C, Milella E, Pallua N. 2005, Implantation of preadipocyte-loaded hyaluronic acid-based scaffolds into nude mice to evaluate potential for soft tissue engineering. *Biomaterials*, 26:7025–7037.

Jansen JA, Dhert WJ, Van der Waerden JP, Von Recum AF. 1994, Semi-quantitative and qualitative histologic analysis method for the evaluation of implant biocompatibility. *J Invest Surg*, 7:123–134.

Katz AJ, Llull R, Hedrick MH, Futrell JW. 1999, Emerging approaches to the tissue engineering of fat. *Clin Plast Surg*, 26:587–603.

Lanza RP, Langer RS, Vacanti J. 2000, *Principles of Tissue Engineering*, Academic Press, San Diego, CA.

Lee AV, Zhang P, Ivanova M, Bonnette S, Oesterreich S, Rosen JM, Grimm S, Hovey RC, Vonderhaar BK, Kahn CR, Torres D. 2003, Developmental and hormonal signals dramatically alter the localization and abundance of insulin receptor substrate proteins in the mammary gland. *Endocrinology*, 144:2683–2694.

McGlohorn JB, Grimes LW, Webster SS, Burg KJ. 2003, Characterization of cellular carriers for use in injectable tissue-engineering composites. *J Biomed Mater Res Part A*, 66:441–449.

Morrison WA, Marre D, Grinsell D, Batty A, Trost N, O'Connor, AJ. 2016, Creation of a large adipose tissue construct in humans using a tissue-engineering chamber: a step forward in the clinical application of soft tissue engineering. *EBioMed*, 6:238–245.

Patrick CW. 2004, Breast tissue engineering. *Annu Rev Biomed Eng*, 6:109–130.

Patrick CW, Jr. 2000, Adipose tissue engineering: the future of breast and soft tissue reconstruction following tumor resection. *Semin Surg Oncol*, 19:302–311.

Patrick CW, Jr. 2001, Tissue engineering strategies for adipose tissue repair. *Anat Rec*, 263:361–366.

Patrick CW, Mikos AG, McIntire LV. 1998, *Frontiers in Tissue Engineering*, Pergamon, Oxford, UK; New York.

Patrick CW, Jr., Uthamanthil R, Beahm E, Frye C. 2008, Animal models for adipose tissue engineering. *Tissue Eng Part B Rev*, 14:167–178.

Peixing WU, Suzuta F, Hikasa Y, Kagota K. 2001, Effects of lipid-related factors on adipocyte differentiation of bovine stromal-vascular cells in primary culture. *J Vet Med Sci*, 62:933–939.

Petrites-Murphy MB. 1992, Mammary carcinoma with peritoneal metastasis in a cow. *Vet Pathol Online*, 29:552–553.

Renneker R, Cutler M. 1952, Psychological problems of adjustment to cancer of the breast. *J Am Med Assoc*, 148:833–838.

Rodbell M. 1964, Metabolism of isolated fat cells. I. Effects of hormones on glucose metabolism and lipolysis. *J Biol Chem*, 239:375–380.

Rowley JA, Madlambayan G, Mooney DJ. 1999, Alginate hydrogels as synthetic extracellular matrix materials. *Biomaterials*, 20:45–53.

Rowson AR, Daniels KM, Ellis SE, Hovey RC. 2012, Growth and development of the mammary glands of livestock: a veritable barnyard of opportunities. *Semin Cell Dev Biol*, 23:557–566.

Russo J, Lynch H, Russo IH. 2001, Mammary gland architecture as a determining factor in the susceptibility of the human breast to cancer. *Breast J*, 7:278–291.

Simonacci F, Bertozzi N, Pio Grieco M, Grignaffini E, Raposio E. 2016, Autologous fat transplantation: a literature review. *Ann Med Surg*, 12:94–100.

Solinas-Toldo S, Lengauer C, Fries R. 1995, Comparative genome map of human and cattle. *Genomics*, 27:489–496.

Thomas CB, Maxson S, Burg KJL. 2011, Preparation and characterization of a composite of demineralized bone matrix fragments and polylactide beads for bone tissue engineering. *J Biomater Sci: Polym Ed*, 22:589–610.

Threadgill DW, Womack JE. 1990, Syntenic conservation between humans and cattle. I. Human chromosome 9. *Genomics*, 8:22–28.

Threadgill DW, Adkison LR, Womack JE. 1990, Syntenic conservation between humans and cattle. II. Human chromosome 12. *Genomics*, 8:29–34.

Třesohlavá E, Popelka S, Machová L, Rypáček F. 2009, Modification of polylactide surfaces with lactide-ethylene oxide functional block copolymers: accessibility of functional groups. *Biomacromolecules*, 11:68–75.

Vierck JL, Dal Porto D, Dodson MV. 2001, Induction of differentiation of adipofibroblasts using a defined treatment medium without DMI. *Basic Appl Myol*, 11:99–104.

Walgenbach KJ, Voigt M, Riabikhin AW, Andree C, Schaefer DJ, Galla TJ, Stark GB. 2001, Tissue engineering in plastic reconstructive surgery. *Anat Record*, 263:372–378.

Wang S, Cui W, Bei J. 2005, Bulk and surface modifications of polylactide. *Anal Bioanal Chem*, 381:547–556.

Womack JE, Kata SR. 1995, Bovine genome mapping: evolutionary inference and the power of comparative genomics. *Curr Opin Genet Dev*, 5(6):725–733.

Young DA, Christman KL. 2012, Injectable biomaterials for adipose tissue engineering. *Biomed Mater*, 7:024104.

CHAPTER 6

Application of Nanoscale Materials for Regenerative Engineering of Musculoskeletal Tissues

Arijit Bhattacharjee*, Garima Lohiya,* Aman Mahajan,* M. Sriram,* and Dhirendra S. Katti

Indian Institute of Technology Kanpur

CONTENTS

---

* Authors contributed equally.

6.1   REGENERATIVE ENGINEERING OF MUSCULOSKELETAL TISSUES

Musculoskeletal tissue injuries are one of the major health burdens affecting millions of people worldwide [1]. Current treatment approaches for musculoskeletal injuries are only partially successful in combatting the tissue injury and its high disease burden. Tissue/regenerative engineering has emerged as a promising approach to repair, restore, and regenerate injured tissues. Tissue engineering aims to do so, using its three primary components – scaffolds, cells, and bioactive factors – either alone or in combinations. Scaffolds act as a transient support for the regeneration of tissues by providing native-like three-dimensional (3D) microenvironments. In this regard, the interaction of scaffold material with the host tissue or cells plays a vital role in determining cell behavior and consequential tissue regeneration. Furthermore, to facilitate tissue regeneration, the choice of appropriate cell types at populations large enough to be effective clinically is necessary to obtain the desired response. Apart from scaffolds and cells, various bioactive growth factors have been extensively used in the regeneration of musculoskeletal tissues. Taken together, regenerative engineering is a very promising approach for the regeneration of injured musculoskeletal tissues. In this chapter, we discuss recent advances in methods of fabrication of nanoscale materials and nanoscale material-based scaffolds, their effect on the regulation of cell behavior, and their use in the regeneration of musculoskeletal tissues.

6.2   NANOSCALE MATERIALS

Musculoskeletal tissues are highly organized tissues with hierarchical structures ranging from nanoscale extracellular matrix components and microscale cells to macroscale tissues. When the musculoskeletal tissues are damaged beyond their own repair capability, external therapeutic interventions are needed to repair and regenerate the lost/damaged tissues. One such intervention is tissue engineering which has emerged as an exciting approach for the regeneration and repair of damaged tissues. Furthermore, recent advances in the field of nanotechnology have led to the development of various nanoscale materials which, when incorporated in conventional tissue engineering scaffolds, helps to better mimic the native structure of tissue and, thus, improve tissue functionality. A material having one or more dimensions of approximately 1–100 nm is termed a nanoscale material [2]. Nanoscale materials differ from their bulk counterparts as they have very small size, very high surface area to volume ratio, tunable chemical and physical properties, and various surface functionalities. These properties of nanomaterials facilitate the development of composite scaffolds which show desired cell–material interaction and make them more suitable for biomedical applications. Nanofibers, nanoparticles, nanotubes/nanorods, nanocomposites, and nanopatterns are some of the nanoscale materials which are discussed in detail in the following sections.

6.3 TYPES OF NANOSCALE MATERIALS AND THEIR EFFECT ON CELL BEHAVIOR

6.3.1 Nanofibers

Nanofibrous scaffolds have been widely used in multiple biomedical applications such as tissue engineering, drug delivery systems, and wound care [3]. Technically, fibers with diameter range of 1–100 nm should be referred to as nanofibers; however, fibers with diameter up to 500 nm are commonly referred to as nanofibers. Nanofibers possess multiple advantages over microfibers, which make them more suitable for biomedical applications. For example, nanofibers have larger surface area to volume ratios, which enables efficient surface functionalization and immobilization of bioactive molecules such as growth factors and drugs to their surface, thereby improving their functionality for use in regenerative engineering [4]. Since the extracellular matrix (ECM) is made up of 3D fibrous meshes of collagen, nanofibrous scaffolds act as physical mimics of the ECM and, hence, are an interesting scaffold system for regenerative engineering. In this section, we will discuss some of the most commonly used techniques for nanofiber fabrication and their influence on the regulation of various cellular functions with special emphasis on their application in regenerative engineering.

6.3.1.1 Methods of Nanofiber Fabrication

The increasing popularity of nanofiber-based scaffolds in regenerative engineering has prompted the need for improved fabrication methods. With mimicking the native ECM as one of the central goals, a fabrication method should have the ability to tune different features of a nanofibrous scaffold like fiber diameter, orientation, and density of fiber mesh. Many techniques including melt blowing, electrospinning, bicomponent spinning, force spinning, flash spinning, phase separation, template synthesis, drawing, etc. have been explored for the fabrication of nanofibers [5]. While each technique has its own advantages and disadvantages, electrospinning is by far the most commonly used and, consequently, well-studied technique. Electrospinning makes use of a high electric potential to draw a continuous fine jet of fiber from a polymer solution or a melt which is then deposited on a grounded collector. The popularity of electrospinning can be attributed to its simplicity and highly flexible nature to produce fibers with different characteristics. Ambient conditions [6], properties of electrospinning solution, and electrospinning process parameters [7] have been shown to influence the properties of the resultant fibers. Therefore, by optimizing these parameters, fibers of desired morphology and orientation can be fabricated. For example, solution viscosity, voltage supplied, and spinneret-to-collector distance can be used to control the nanofiber diameter. Nanofibers with diameter ranging from as low as ~2 nm [8] to as high as a few microns can be fabricated by varying only a few parameters. Moreover, the collector can be modified to obtain aligned fibers that mimic organized ECM present in tissues such as tendons, ligaments, and neural tissue [9–11]. However, the conventional electrospinning apparatus is not easily scalable and, hence, is limited to laboratory scale applications. To overcome this limitation, various modification to the conventional electrospinning process has been performed in recent years, which include multiple jet electrospinning, multiple needle electrospinning, needleless electrospinning, and dual electrospinning [5]. Apart from this, several pre- and post-fabrication modifications have enabled fabrication of nanofibers with better characteristics required for different end applications. Such modifications include coaxial electrospinning [12], multilayered electrospinning [13], electrospinning-co-electrospraying [14], and blending [15], which have led to improvement in the characteristics of nanofibers. However, drawbacks such as inability to form 3D scaffold, toxicity of the solvents used, and use of high voltage have necessitated the search for alternative nanofiber fabrication techniques. In this regard, force-spinning technique which uses centrifugal force to draw fibers from the spinneret is currently gaining momentum. When compared to the electrospinning technique, force-spinning provided a significant improvement in the productivity of nanofibers [16]. However, additional studies are needed to fully evaluate the potential of force-spinning for the fabrication of nanofibers.

6.3.1.2 Effects of Nanofibers on Cell Behavior

Since nanofibers can be considered as a physical mimic of native ECM components of various musculoskeletal tissues, many studies have investigated the role of nanofibers in the regulation of cell fate processes. A recent study showed that cell behavior in synthetic fibrillar networks was similar to that observed in collagen matrix [17]. This indicated that fibrillar scaffolds could be a better model to study cell behavior than the conventionally used elastic hydrogel systems [17]. Furthermore, various studies have demonstrated that cells respond to changes in physical properties of nanofibrous scaffolds such as fiber diameter, orientation, and stiffness.

Recently, it has been demonstrated that aligned fibers alone promote stem cell differentiation into specific lineages. For example, mesenchymal stem cells (MSCs) cultured on aligned fibers expressed tendon specific markers like scleraxis, collagen type 1, and decorin significantly higher than MSCs cultured on random fibers. The ECM deposition was also along the direction of fiber alignment, which is of significance in engineering tissues with highly organized ECM like tendon [18]. Similarly, aligned fibers have also been shown to influence cell migration. In a recent study, Shang et al. have demonstrated that the migration efficiency of rat periodontal ligament cells was three-fold higher on aligned fibers than their migration efficiency on random fibers [19]. Several recent studies have elucidated the influence of fiber diameter on cell proliferation and differentiation [20, 21]. Apart from this, fiber diameter has been shown to influence cell alignment on oriented nanofibers. Whited and Rylander demonstrated that primary human umbilical vein endothelial cells (HUVEC), when cultured on 100 and 300 nm electrospun aligned fibers, aligned along the fibers but the cell alignment was not observed on 1,200 nm fibers [22]. A recent study to investigate the effect of fiber stiffness on cell behavior showed that cells cultured on soft fibers, because of cellular contractile force, were able to recruit soft fibers but not stiff fibers toward themselves. This fiber recruitment increased the ECM ligand density at cell's vicinity, enhancing focal adhesion formation and thereby cell proliferation [17]. Taken together, nanofibrous scaffolds due to their resemblance to ECM of natural tissues have a considerable impact on various cell fate processes, which, in turn, greatly influences repair and regeneration of damaged tissues. The cell behavior on nanofibers is sensitive not only to the physical properties of the fibers but also to the chemical composition, surface properties (charge and hydro-philicity/-phobicity), and cell type used. Therefore, appropriate optimization of parameters needs to be performed to elicit suitable cellular response which will eventually lead to functional tissue regeneration.

6.3.2 Nanoparticles

Tissue engineering focuses on the repair, restoration, and regeneration of complex tissues and organs which often require the sustained presence of bioactive molecules that facilitate different cell functions such as proliferation and differentiation. This sustained presence can be achieved via localized delivery of appropriate bioactive molecules by encapsulating them in nanoparticles (NPs). The NPs, in turn, can be incorporated in a scaffold for site-specific delivery. Incorporating the NPs in scaffolds has a two-fold advantage: (i) improvement in mechanical properties of composite scaffolds and (ii) sustained delivery of the encapsulated bioactive molecule. Therefore, NP-based bioactive molecule delivery has become an important approach in bioactive molecule-mediated tissue engineering strategies. Apart from this, NPs alone can direct cell fate processes. A material with all three dimensions at the nanoscale (<100 nm) is termed a 'nanoparticle.' However, as in the case of nanofiber, submicron particles are commonly referred to as NPs. The advances in nanotechnology have led to the development of various kinds of nanoparticulate delivery vehicles such as polymeric NPs, metallic NPs, non-metallic NPs, micellar NPs, liposomal NPs, and dendrimers, of which some of the important ones will be discussed in the next section.

6.3.2.1 Methods of Nanoparticle Fabrication

Advancements in the field of nanotechnology have led to the development of various methods for the synthesis of nanoparticles with specific characteristics such as shape and size. Recently, advanced methods for synthesis of monodisperse polystyrene NPs with mean diameter less than 100 nm have been proposed via aqueous emulsion polymerization using an amphoteric initiator 2,2'-azobis[N-(2-carboxyethyl)-2-methylpropionamidine] (VA-057) and sub millimolar concentration of an anionic surfactant [23]. Another study reported synthesis of size-tunable polymeric NPs by an advanced nanoprecipitation method, which involves 3D hydrodynamic flow focused in single-layer microchannel [24]. A uniform and narrow size distribution of NPs is a key prerequisite for their role as efficient delivery vehicles. Superparamagnetic iron oxide nanoparticles (SPIONS) have been widely explored for their application in the diagnosis and treatment (hyperthermia) of cancer. Owing to easy agglomeration of SPIONs, recent research focused on surface modification of SPIONs with biocompatible materials such as silica, gold, citric acid, and polyethylene glycol to prevent their agglomeration and maintain their monodispersity [25]. Furthermore, advances in the synthesis of shape-controlled noble metal NPs by radiolysis route have been reported [26]. In addition to these, bimetallic NPs consisting of magnetic NPs and noble metal NPs are gaining importance owing to their immense potential in many fields including catalysis, biosensing, and biomedical applications. For example, there are studies which focus on the synthesis of AuAg nanostructures by using tyrosine or poly(ethylene oxide)-poly(propylene oxide) as a reducing agent [27]. Likewise, there is an increased interest in the development of core-shell NPs. For example, smart core-shell hybrid nanogels with Ag nanoparticle core and poly(N-isopropylacrylamide-co-acrylic acid) shell have been fabricated using the method of copolymerization [28, 29]. Thus, various kinds of NPs with controlled shape, size, and surface functionality enabling site-specific and local delivery of biomolecules/cargo are in development to facilitate tissue regeneration.

6.3.2.2 Effect of Nanoparticles on Cell Behavior

Surface topography and chemical modification of substrates have been known to mediate cell behavior. Various scaffolds incorporating NPs, such as poly(lactide-co-glycolide) nanoparticles (PLGA NP) incorporated chitosan-gelatin scaffolds and polyurethane NP incorporated gelatin scaffolds, have been fabricated to study the effect of change in surface topography on various cell fate processes, such as differentiation, migration, proliferation, adhesion, and apoptosis. Many studies showed that nano-roughness of substrates imparted by NPs affect cellular processes in a cell-specific manner [30]. However, the results suggest that change in physical properties of scaffolds due to the incorporation of NPs did not alter cell viability and cell adhesion onto scaffolds [31, 32]. It has been found that NP-modified surfaces can direct differentiation of human mesenchymal stem cells into specific lineages [33–35]. Balasundaram et al. reported a composite scaffold made of hydroxyapatite NPs and calcium phosphate that promoted osteoblast adhesion and growth [36]. In another study, it was demonstrated that dexamethasone-loaded dendrimer NPs encapsulated in scaffolds enhanced the osteogenic differentiation of murine bone marrow stromal cells [37]. Taken together, these results suggest that NP incorporated scaffolds can be suitably used to facilitate tissue regeneration. In another application, silver NP-incorporated scaffolds have been used as biocompatible antimicrobial bone grafts wherein the silver NPs provided antimicrobial properties without affecting the ability of scaffolds to promote cell (osteoblasts) proliferation [38]. Apart from this, a recent study demonstrated that NP-incorporated scaffolds can also be used for *in situ* differentiation of MSCs into multiple lineages within a single implant. In this study, different small-interfering RNAs (siRNAs) NPs were immobilized into scaffolds which enabled spatially controlled release of siRNAs and, thus, mediated the differentiation of MSCs into different lineages [39]. Another study reported that NPs such as SPIONs could independently promote human mesenchymal stem cells (hMSCs) proliferation [40].

Cellular uptake of NPs is a prerequisite for the use of NPs in some biomedical applications and size of NPs is one of the important properties which regulates NP–cell interaction [41]. Shi et al. showed that among three sizes (20, 40, and 80 nm) of hydroxyapatite (HA) NPs, 20 nm HA NPs showed the highest retardation of osteosarcoma growth and supported viability and proliferation of hMSCs [42]. Apart from size, cellular uptake of NPs is controlled by NP surface charge and hydrophobicity. It has been found that cationic NPs, in general, are more cytotoxic than anionic NPs due to their ability to cause more marked disruption of cell membrane integrity and stronger lysosomal and mitochondrial damage than anionic NPs. Studies also suggested that non-phagocytic cells take up cationic NPs to a greater extent, whereas phagocytic cells favorably take up anionic NPs [43]. Also, it has been found that particles with larger aspect ratios have higher internalization rates and impact on different cellular behavior like proliferation, adhesion, cytoskeleton formation, migration, and apoptosis [44]. Thus, when cells encounter any nanomaterial, they exhibit different responses based on the identity of NPs and its microenvironment. Therefore, having proper understanding of NP–cell interaction and factors affecting this interaction will significantly help in the successful application of NPs in tissue regeneration.

6.3.3 Nanotubes

Nanotubes are 2D nanomaterials having diameter in the nanometer scale and long cylindrical shape with large inner volumes having structural similarity to tiny drinking straws. Because of their distinct inner and outer surface properties, nanotubes can be functionalized with various groups such as hydroxyl, carboxyl, and alkyl chains [45]. Due to their distinct mechanical, chemical, electrical, and biological properties, nanotubes are considered an exciting material for scaffold modification in the engineering of a wide range of tissues, including musculoskeletal tissues. Nanotubes used in scaffolds for musculoskeletal tissue regeneration are mostly synthesized using inorganic, metallic, and polymeric materials such as carbon, boron nitride, titanium dioxide, glass, and chitin.

6.3.3.1 Methods of Nanotube Fabrication

A wide variety of methods have been developed to fabricate nanotubes to meet the requirement of musculoskeletal tissue regeneration. Carbon nanotubes (CNTs) are the most widely used nanotubes for musculoskeletal regeneration, which are fabricated from either single or concentric rolled graphene sheets, and are known as single-walled carbon nanotubes and multi-walled carbon nanotubes, respectively. Commonly used methods for fabrication of CNTs include: (i) arc–discharge, (ii) laser ablation, and (iii) chemical vapor deposition (CVD) [46, 47]. Among these, CVD is the most widely used method for synthesis of CNTs. CVD utilizes carbon source in gas phase and an energy source to transfer energy to the carbon molecules. For this, hydrocarbons are used as a carbon source which flow through a quartz tube placed inside an oven (~720°C), which produces pure carbon molecules. These carbon molecules diffuse and move toward the substrate where it binds to form a nanotube-like structure. Unlike laser ablation and arc–discharge method which involve a high-processing temperature of over 1,700°C and little control over the structural integrity of nanotubes, CVD is a relatively low temperature method (<800°C) with better control over nanotube length, diameter, alignment, purity, and orientation. Additionally, CVD offers other advantages such as cost-effective and large-scale fabrication of CNTs.

Recently, metallic nanotubes like titanium dioxide (TiO_2) and zirconium dioxide nanotubes have gained importance in musculoskeletal tissue engineering applications due to their good biocompatibility, excellent tensile strength, and good corrosion resistance. Metallic nanotubes are fabricated using methods such as electrochemical anodic oxidation, assisted-templating, and hydrothermal treatment [48]. Among these, electrochemical anodic oxidation method has low cost and improved control on the dimensions of the nanotubes, and is applicable to a wide range of metals. In this method, nanotubes are produced by a process called anodization, which is electrolytic passivation of the metal to form a metal oxide layer on the base material. Dimensions of the nanotubes produced using electrochemical anodic oxidation can be controlled by varying electrolyte composition/pH, voltage, and anodizing time. Recently, TiO_2 nanotubes were grown on nanograined substrates using a combination of surface mechanical attrition treatment (SMAT) and anodization. It was observed that the SMATed–anodized samples had larger diameter and length compared to the non-SMATed samples [49]. Apart from inorganic and metallic nanotubes, polymeric nanotubes have also been explored for musculoskeletal tissue engineering applications and have been synthesized using both natural and synthetic polymers such as chitin/chitosan, nylon 6, poly(3, 4-ethylene dioxythiophene), and polystyrene. The methods commonly used for the fabrication of polymeric nanotubes include (i) electrospinning, (ii) membrane templating, (iii) layer-by-layer processing, and (iv) *in situ* polymerization. Although all methods have their own advantages and disadvantages, the membrane templating method is the most widely studied, effective, and simple method for the fabrication of nanotubes [50]. Byun et al. designed a template by allowing adhesion of anodized aluminum oxide (AAO), synthesized by two-step anodization, over various modified polymeric layers to achieve a high-density array of freestanding and vertically aligned nanotubes. However, these templates have yet to be explored in the field of tissue engineering [51]. Electrospun nanotubes have been prepared from electrospun nanofibers using cryostat microtome in conjunction with probe tip sonication while layer-by-layer fabrication process involves concentric alternating layers of polymeric materials [52]. Chapman et al. investigated the self-assembly of peptide-polymer conjugates into nanotubes and demonstrated that β-sheet networks of peptides conjugated to polymer guide the formation of nanotubes [53]. Taken together, the material, method, and parameters of fabrication govern the type and dimensions of fabricated nanotubes.

6.3.3.2 Effect of Nanotubes on Cell Behavior

Cell fate processes like cell adhesion, migration, proliferation, and differentiation depend on nanotopography and microenvironment of substrate that provide external cues, which, in turn, direct cell signaling and gene expression. There are numerous studies that have investigated the impact of nanotube diameter, length, alignment, and surface density of nanotube networks on cell behavior. A recent study demonstrated that cells attached more on TiO_2 nanotubes grown on nanograined substrates than on coarse grained substrates; however, cell spreading on these nanotubes was relatively lower due to space inhibition mechanism [49]. In another study, Brammer et al. investigated cell migration on nanostructured nanotube surface and flat nanotube surface. The results showed enhanced cell migration and actin filament formation on nanostructured surface when compared to flat nanotube [54]. In another study, it was observed that the addition of halloysite nanotubes to alginate or chitosan hydrogels created a cell supportive environment for mesenchymal stem cells and pre-osteoblasts to proliferate and differentiate [55]. Furthermore, the alignment in CNT networks allows hMSCs to recognize individual CNTs in CNT network which further allows control over growth direction and differentiation of hMSCs compared to the random networks of nanotubes. The hMSCs on aligned CNT network allowed enhanced osteogenic differentiation compared to hMSCs on random CNT network. The study also showed that the surface density of aligned nanotube networks significantly influenced cell alignment [56]. Similarly, MSC proliferation, motility, and differentiation have been shown to be influenced by the diameter of nanotubes. In this regard, Park et al. investigated the effect of nanotube diameter on the differentiation of MSCs. The results from the study revealed that MSCs showed enhanced differentiation into osteoclasts on nanotube with the diameter of 15 nm than nanotube with the diameter of 100 nm [57]. Another study observed that nanotube diameter of 70 nm is optimal for osteogenic differentiation of human adipose-derived stem cells [58]. Therefore, nanotubes can be used in the modification of scaffolding systems to enable enhanced cell attachment, proliferation, differentiation, and synthesis of tissue-specific matrix for functional regeneration of musculoskeletal tissue.

6.3.4 Nanopatterns

Structurally, the ECM of various tissues like bone, muscle, and heart consists of highly oriented patterned structures with nanoscale dimensions [59]. Taking this ultrastructural feature as an inspiration, the development of ECM mimicking nanopatterned scaffolds has been an attractive strategy for the regeneration of various musculoskeletal tissues. Therefore, the fabrication of biomimetic nanopatterned substrates with suitable physical or chemical cues to modulate cell fate processes has been extensively explored in tissue regeneration.

6.3.4.1 Methods of Nanopattern Fabrication

Fabrication techniques used for nanopatterning of matrices for regenerative engineering applications include photolithography, electron beam lithography, dip-pen lithography, nano-imprint lithography, capillary force lithography, colloidal lithography, etc. [60, 61]. These techniques are associated with inherent advantages and disadvantages; however, photolithography and electron beam lithography are the most widely used methods for fabrication of nanopatterned substrates for musculoskeletal tissue regeneration. In this process, geometric shapes on a mask are transferred to the surface of a silicon wafer. The major steps of nanopattern fabrication using photolithographic technique include cleaning of silicon wafer, formation of barrier layer, photoresist application, soft-baking, alignment of mask, exposure and development of pattern, and finally, hard-baking [60]. Electron beam lithography uses electron beam to cleave the unmasked region of the substrate leading to the formation of desired pattern [60]. Apart from these two techniques, another versatile lithography technique is the dip-pen nanolithography (DPN) technique that uses atomic force microscopy tip to pattern molecules of interest on a substrate in a specified pattern with nanometer scale precision [62].

All the aforementioned nano-fabrication techniques help improve our understanding of the effect of nanoscale features of substrate on cell behavior and, thereby, facilitate tissue regeneration.

6.3.4.2 Effect of Nanopatterns on Cell Behavior

It has been demonstrated that the ECM nanotopography plays a crucial role in the regulation of cell behavior [63]. The substrates that mimic ECM nanotopography have been shown to influence morphology, adhesion, migration, proliferation, reprogramming, and differentiation of cells, thereby regulating tissue repair and regeneration [63].

In a recent study, Kim et al. demonstrated that spacing of nanogrooves can control different fate processes like adhesion, migration, and differentiation of hMSCs into osteogenic or neurogenic lineage, indicating that nanotopographical density can be taken advantage of for the design of scaffolds for regenerative medicine [64]. In another study, hMSCs cultured on Arg-Gly-Asp (RGD) micro-/nanopatterned substrates with different nano-spacing have demonstrated RGD nano-spacing to be a robust regulator of stem cell differentiation into osteogenic and adipogenic lineages [65]. Similarly, there are several other studies which demonstrate that nanopatterned surfaces can efficiently regulate cell differentiation [66–68].

Apart from the regulation of adhesion, proliferation, and differentiation, patterned substrates have also been shown to influence cell reprogramming. Downing et al. have demonstrated that cells cultured on grooved matrices undergo enhanced reprogramming and can replace the requirement of chemical epigenetic modifiers [69]. In the future, control of cell behavior by nanotopography might provide improved understanding of various signaling pathways and cell functions, which, in turn, can be taken advantage of in tissue engineering applications.

6.3.5 Nanocomposites

A single material is most often unable to meet the complex requirements of a scaffold for repair and regeneration of damaged musculoskeletal tissues. To meet this challenge, multiphase materials that combine the advantages of individual components have been designed. Nanocomposites are an example of such materials with the discontinuous phase of the composite having nanoscale size (1–100 nm) in at least one of its dimensions [70].

6.3.5.1 Methods of Nanocomposite Fabrication

For the fabrication of nanocomposites, it is important to select a suitable discontinuous phase material that will provide required physical, chemical, and biological cues necessary for tissue regeneration. Various methods either alone or in combination have been employed in the fabrication of nanocomposites for regenerative engineering of musculoskeletal tissues, which include electrospinning, 3D printing, layer-by-layer self-assembly, solvent casting, freeze drying, electrodeposition, and *in situ* polymerization [71]. Among these, electrospinning and 3D printing are the most widely used methods for the fabrication of nanocomposites.

Electrospinning has been discussed in detail as a method of nanofiber fabrication; however, it is also commonly used for the fabrication of nanocomposites. The procedure is similar, except in this case, both the constituents are electrospun together to obtain the nanocomposite fibers.

In the recent past, use of 3D printing for the fabrication of nanocomposite scaffolds has gained momentum. It is a versatile technique which provides rapid fabrication with precise control over pore architecture and dimensions of fabricated scaffolds. In this technique, scaffolds are created using layer-by-layer deposition of bioink (polymers, ceramics, etc.) and a computer-aided model [72]. The most widely used 3D printing methods for the fabrication of tissue engineering composite scaffolds include vat photo-polymerization method, fused filament fabrication method, selective laser sintering method, and inkjet 3D printing [72]. Although 3D printed nanocomposite scaffolds offer several advantages like patient-specific scaffold design, rapid fabrication, and precise control on architecture, the number of available bioprinting materials are limited. Such limitations can be overcome by the development of newer and better bioinks and combining 3D printing techniques with other scaffold fabrication methods for the synthesis of multifunctional nanocomposite scaffolds.

6.3.5.2 Effect of Nanocomposites on Cell Behavior

In recent years, various nanocomposite scaffolds have been shown to influence cell fate processes that are central to tissue engineering applications. It has been demonstrated that nano-cues can modulate various signaling pathways, thereby affecting cell fate processes. This has led to an increased interest in the development of nanocomposite scaffolds for regenerative engineering of musculoskeletal tissues.

The composition of nanocomposite scaffolds often influences their effect on cell behavior, including adhesion, proliferation, and differentiation. In a recent study, Lee et al. demonstrated that reduced graphene oxide/nano-hydroxyapatite (nHAp) nanocomposite significantly enhanced the osteogenic differentiation of MC3T3-E1 cells in vitro. Furthermore, this nanocomposite graft also led to increased new bone formation in rabbit full-thickness calvarial defects after 4 weeks of implantation [73].

In another recent study, Barlas et al. demonstrated that folic acid modified clay/polymer nanocomposites selectively enhanced the adhesion and proliferation of HeLa cells [74]. Furthermore, it has also been demonstrated using chitosan (continuous phase) and poly-methylmethacrylate (discontinuous phase) nanocomposite that bone marrow-derived MSCs can be differentiated to osteogenic lineage [75]. Similarly, several other studies have demonstrated that the incorporation of nHAp in the scaffold system also significantly enhanced osteogenic differentiation of MSCs [76, 77].

Furthermore, using nanocomposite hydrogels composed of periodic mesoporous organosilica (PMO)/alginate, Seda Kehr and Riehemann demonstrated that cell migration (3T3 and C-6 glioma) is directly proportional to the concentration of PMO [78]. However, the effect of PMOs on cell growth is cell type-specific as higher concentration of PMOs reduced the C-6 glioma cell growth although growth of 3T3 cells enhanced with increasing concentration of PMOs. In another study, Bhowmick et al. fabricated a

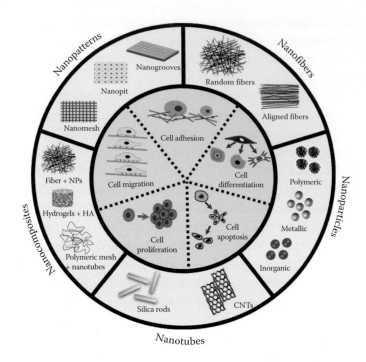

FIGURE 6.1   Effect of nanoscale materials, such as nanoparticles, nanofibers, nanopatterns, nano-composites, and nanotubes, on cell behavior.

biomimetic nanocomposite-based scaffold (mimicking complex bone architecture) and demonstrated that the nanocomposite scaffold enhanced the proliferation of osteosarcoma cells *in vitro* [79]. Taken together, nanocomposite scaffolds offer mechanical, chemical, and biological support to cells, and this effect is dependent on the nanoscale interaction of scaffolds with host tissues. These interactions play a crucial role in mediating various cell fate processes like adhesion, migration, proliferation, and differentiation and, hence, can be tuned to facilitate the process of musculoskeletal tissue regeneration [80] (Figure 6.1).

6.4 NANOSCALE MATERIALS IN MUSCULOSKELETAL TISSUE ENGINEERING

In the previous section, we discussed methods of fabrication of different nanoscale materials and their effect on various cell fate processes. In this section, we will discuss the application of these nanoscale materials in regeneration of various musculoskeletal tissues, namely, cartilage, bone, ligament/tendon, and muscles.

6.4.1 Cartilage

Articular cartilage, a load-bearing connective tissue, is subjected to various injuries during its lifetime. However, since cartilage tissue is avascular and is sparsely populated with progenitor cells, its ability to regenerate is limited. To regenerate damaged cartilage, tissue engineering has emerged as a new approach that makes use of different types of nano-materials (nanofibers, nanocomposites, etc.) for cartilage regeneration. In a recent study.

Liu et al. demonstrated the capability of self-assembled nanofibrous hollow microspheres fabricated using star-shaped poly(L-lactic acid) to regenerate hyaline cartilage in a rabbit osteochondral defect model [81]. These hollow microspheres showed stable integration with the host cartilage and enhanced cartilage matrix deposition when compared to polyethylene glycol hydrogels and chondrocytes suspension only indicating that the cartilage matrix deposition was due to the nanofibrous nature of the scaffolds used [81]. The geometrical topography, particularly at the nanometer length scale, have been shown to affect mesenchymal stem cell differentiation into chondrocytes. Recently, it was observed that nanopatterns, namely, nano-grill and nano-holes, synthesized on polycaprolactone surface via thermal nanoimprinting resulted in improved mesenchymal stem cell aggregation, differentiation, and cytoskeletal remodeling, thus facilitating hyaline cartilage formation compared to non-topographical patterns [82]. Apart from nanofibers and nanopatterns, nanocomposites which closely mimic the complex architectural properties of native tissue have been commonly used for tissue regeneration. Since cartilage is a complex tissue, therefore, nanocomposites based on polymers in combination with other nanomaterials have been considered for its regeneration. Chahine et al. observed that nanocomposite of agarose and SWCNTs functionally modified with carboxyl groups (COOH) demonstrated increased expression of collagen type 2a and aggrecan (cartilage-specific markers) when compared to control groups that were without SWCNTs. This observation was attributed to the negative charge of COOH groups on SWCNTs, which mimics proteoglycans present in native cartilage matrix [83]. In addition to the aforementioned nanostructures, nanoparticles have been explored for cartilage regeneration applications. They have been extensively studied as a drug delivery vehicle at the defect site for tissue regeneration. Kartogenin, a small molecular compound, has been shown to have chondrogenic effects on bone marrow-derived mesenchymal stem cells and synovium derived mesenchymal stem cells. Taking advantage of these properties, Shi et al. demonstrated that kartogenin-loaded poly(lactide-co-glycolide) nanoparticles impregnated in photocross-linked ultraviolet light hyaluronic acid scaffolds facilitated hyaline cartilage regeneration in an osteochondral rabbit model [84]. Collectively, these studies show implications of the nanomaterials in the regeneration of cartilage defects.

6.4.2 Bone

Human bone is composed of organic and inorganic components having a hierarchical structure with built-in nanoscale to microscale dimensional architecture. Due to this, several nanoscale materials have been extensively used as bone ECM mimics like nanofibers, nanoparticles, nanopatterns, nanotubes, and nanocomposites. Native bone architecture can be closely mimicked by these nanostructured scaffolds which, in turn, can regulate cell fate processes like proliferation, migration, and differentiation, leading to the formation of functional tissue. In this section, we discuss recent advances in the use of nanostructures for bone regeneration.

Nanofibers are one of the most widely used nanostructures for bone tissue engineering as they offer several advantages like tunable mechanical and surface properties, delivery of bioactive molecules, and ease of fabrication of ECM mimetic structures [85]. Apart from the use of conventional nanofibers (including blends and composites) as bone tissue engineering scaffolds [86–89], recent advancements in this field include the use of core-shell nanofibers, hollow nanofibers, and multilayered nanofibers. In a recent study, Kwak et al. fabricated PLGA collagen multilayered scaffolds using alternate electrospinning and demonstrated that the fabricated scaffold enhanced *in vitro* differentiation of MC3T3-E1 cells [90]. Similarly, core-shell PLGA/collagen nanofibers have been used to investigate the role of recombinant fibronectin and cadherin on adhesion and differentiation of hMSCs. The results obtained from this study demonstrated that the recombinant protein-loaded core-shell nanofiber scaffold enhanced *in vitro* proliferation and osteogenic differentiation of hMSCs [91].

Another class of widely used nanoscale material systems for bone tissue engineering includes nanocomposites. The nHAp containing nanocomposites are the most extensively studied nanocomposite systems for bone regeneration. However, in recent years, nanocomposites of other materials are also gaining importance for bone regenerative applications. In one such study, Bhowmick et al. synthesized montmorillonite and nHAp-modified zirconium doped chitosan nanocomposite and demonstrated that the developed scaffold was cytocompatible [79]. In another study, calcium/copper-releasing nanocomposite scaffold was shown to induce osteogenic differentiation of rat bone marrow-derived MSCs [92]. Other nanoscale materials such as nanoparticle [93, 94], nanopattern [95, 96], and nanotubes [97, 98] are also being exploited either alone or in combination with macroscale materials as composite scaffold for bone tissue engineering.

6.4.3 Ligament and Tendon

Ligament and tendon injuries are very common musculoskeletal defects that significantly compromise the patient's normal movements and activities. Although surgery is the current gold standard treatment strategy for ligament and tendon injuries, they are associated with certain disadvantages, such as donor site morbidity (autologous reconstruction surgery) and high failure rates (synthetic grafts and allografts) [99]. Tissue engineering of damaged ligament and tendon is considered a potential alternative to reconstruction surgery. Many advancements in tissue engineering strategies, especially in scaffold fabrication, have been made in the last decade for regeneration of damaged ligament and tendon [100]. Ligaments/tendons have a structure-to-function relationship; hence, one of the strategies in ligament/tendon tissue engineering involves the fabrication of scaffolds that mimic the tissue's structure to facilitate regeneration. Recently, use of nanotechnology in scaffold fabrication has led to a significant advancement in the fabrication of nano-structured scaffolds, especially in nanofiber and nanocomposite fabrication. One such study reported a wet-spun biodegradable silk fibroin scaffold with a hierarchical structure involving nanofibrils, microfibers, and fiber bundles for anterior cruciate ligament (ACL) regeneration. The fabricated scaffold had mechanical properties that were comparable to native ACL tissue, indicating its potential for application in ACL tissue engineering [101]. In another study, a micro-/nanofiber hybrid scaffold was assessed for its application in ligament/tendon tissue engineering. Poly(3-hydroxybutyrate) or polycaprolactone nanofibers were electrospun on silk fibroin microfibers and these microfibers were twisted together to make a robust scaffold. The hybrid scaffolds possessed better mechanical properties than silk fibroin fibers and were also cytocompatible to L929 fibroblasts [102]. In a recent study, nanofiber sheets were rolled into nanofiber bundles to mimic the fascicles of ligament tissues [103]. The nanofiber sheets and bundles showed better mechanical properties than their random counterparts, and modification of using aligned nanofiber sheets to form aligned nanofiber bundles improved their yield stresses and yield strains by 107% and 140%, respectively [103]. Apart from nanofibers, nanocomposites have also been investigated for ligament/tendon tissue engineering. A recent study has reported a collagen-based bio-nanocomposite that is reinforced with cellulose nanofibers [104]. The composite cross-linked with genipin exhibited mechanical properties comparable to native ligament/tendon under simulated body conditions even after irradiating it with 25 KGy gamma rays [104]. Another composite material consisting of electrospun polyurethane fibers reinforced with MWCNTs showed good potential to be used as ligament/tendon grafts. The tensile stress of the polyurethane fibers increased from 11.40 to 51.25 MPa, which further increased to 72.78 MPa on aligning the fibers [105]. Empson et al. studied nanoparticles with high elastic modulus for the treatment of sub-failure connective tissue matrix damage [106]. In this study, carbon nano horns injected into injured porcine digitorum tendon infiltrated well into the tissue and improved its elastic modulus significantly when compared to untreated control. Furthermore, in the same study, cellulose nanocrystals improved the cellular activities of tenocytes *in vitro* which was determined using water soluble tetrazolium salt assay [106]. Iannone et al. recently demonstrated that surfaces with nanopatterns can be used to generate 3D human embryonic tendon-like tissues without any added growth factors or exogenous scaffold matrices [107]. Finally, a scaffold used for ligament/tendon tissue engineering should integrate properly with bone to ensure long-term function of the scaffold. In this regard, a recent study fabricated a tri-component scaffold with bone insertion regions made of porous poly(1,8-octanediol-co-citric acid)–hydroxyapatite nanocomposites at both ends of a poly(L-lactide) scaffold for ACL reconstruction. The scaffold integrated well with rabbit bones and showed good tissue ingrowth *in vivo* [108]. Taken together, ligament/tendon tissue engineering has significantly benefited from the advances made in nanomaterial-based strategies, especially in scaffold fabrication.

6.4.4 Muscle

Muscle tissue in mammals is of three types, namely, skeletal muscle, smooth muscle, and cardiac muscle. Skeletal muscles support movement of the body, smooth muscles line internal organs like gastrointestinal tract, and cardiac muscles form muscles of the heart. Conditions such as tumor ablation and burn injuries lead to loss of large amounts of skeletal muscle tissue. Limited availability of host muscle tissue and donor site morbidity limits restoration of lost tissue. As a consequence, tissue engineering of muscles has emerged as an exciting alternative for regeneration and restoration of lost tissue. Several tissue engineering attempts are now being made to develop a muscle construct which can mimic natural tissue, to a large extent, through the development of biomimetic scaffolds. A variety of biomaterials, such as collagen, polycaprolactone, poly(lactic-co-glycolic) acid, and chitosan, are being explored as scaffolding materials for muscle tissue engineering. Studies using scaffolds suggest that providing contact guidance to myoblasts is an essential prereq-uisite for their elongation and alignment [109–112]. In a recent study, Aviss et al. fabricated electrospun PLGA fibrous scaffolds which provided an appropriate topology for myoblast adhesion, elongation, and differentiation in the absence of any additional biochemical sig-naling molecules [113]. In another study, the influence of various types of CNTs on muscle cell response was investigated [114]. The results from this study showed that in the pres-ence of all types of CNTs, intense myoblast proliferation and differentiation into myocytes were observed. Furthermore, in another study, polyethylene glycol-linked multi-walled carbon nanotube films having high hydrophilicity and nanoscale surface roughness have been shown to direct skeletal myogenic differentiation of hMSCs in the absence of myo-genic induction factors [115]. Similarly, another study demonstrated that 3D electroactive graphene foams promoted growth and differentiation of myoblast into functional myo-tubes [116]. Recently, CuO–nanofibrillar cellulose/glycerol based hyperbranched epoxy nanocomposite was validated as a high-performance, biodegradable, and antimicrobial scaffold material for reconstruction of muscle tissues [117]. These and many other studies suggested that topographical cues and electroactivity of scaffolds direct stem cell differen-tiation into myogenic lineage [109, 111]. The development of such 3D platforms can prove to be promising materials for the repair and regeneration of muscle tissue.

Self-regeneration of cardiac muscle is limited due to poor regenerative potential of cardiomyocytes. Tissue engineering-based approach of delivering functional cells to the injured myocardium is one of the methods to overcome the limited repair capability of car-diomyocytes. In an attempt to obtain cardiomyocytes from MSCs, Mooney et al. performed a study in which they showed that electrical stimulation of CNTs provided cardiomimetic cue to MSCs [118]. In another study, Chen et al. demonstrated that biomimetic collagen-chitosan nanofibrous scaffolds promoted the proliferation of both smooth muscle cells and endothelial cells and, hence, could find use in muscle tissue engineering applications [119]. In addition to the aforementioned nanostructures, nanoparticles have also been explored in muscle tissue regeneration. A recent study reported the use of a nanoparticulate system capable of targeting the infarcted heart, which could be useful in delivering a therapeutic agent to the infarcted heart, thereby increasing the local therapeutic dose of the medication and reducing its systemic toxicity [120]. Another study showed that in addition to the tar-geted delivery, nanoparticles could be simultaneously used for imaging, thereby improving the nanoparticles-based treatment modality for ischemia treatment [121].

Overall, since one of the central goals of tissue engineering is the creation of ECM mim-icking scaffolds, the application of nanotechnology helps to mimic or replicate the natural hierarchy of tissue structures and has, hence, opened new realms of advancements in the field of using nanostructures for musculoskeletal tissue regeneration. However, most of the current studies are limited to laboratories and extensive preclinical and clinical studies are required for their successful translation into the clinic (Figure 6.2).

6.5 SUMMARY

In this chapter, we discussed nanoscale scaffold systems commonly used in the regen-eration of injured musculoskeletal tissues. To better understand the role of nanoscale

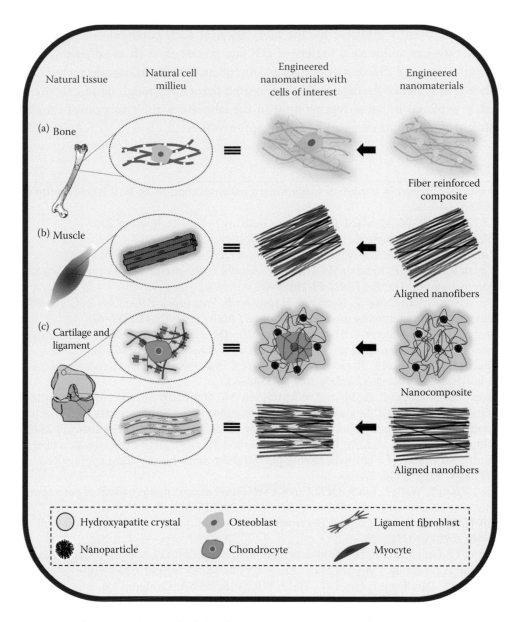

FIGURE 6.2   Schematic of musculoskeletal tissue engineering using biomimetic nanoscale materials. (a) Fiber-reinforced nanocomposite scaffolds that promote osteogenesis, (b) aligned fibrous scaffolds that promote myogenesis, and (c) nanocomposite scaffolds that promote chondrogenesis and aligned fibrous scaffolds that promote ligamentogenesis.

scaffold system-based tissue regeneration, we first discussed the methods of fabrication of various nanoscale materials and how they regulate various cell behavior. Furthermore, we highlighted the use of these materials in the regeneration of specific musculoskeletal tissues.

Nanofibers, nanoparticles, nanotubes, nanopatterns, and nanocomposites are the most prevalent nanoscale materials for musculoskeletal tissue engineering. Various versatile methods are currently available for the fabrication of such nanoscale materials. All of these materials can influence a variety of cell fate processes, such as adhesion, proliferation, migration, and differentiation. As a consequence, these nanoscale materials have been shown to enhance the regeneration of injured tissues. Although nanoscale materials are widely explored in tissue regeneration in the laboratory, their successful translation into clinical applications warrants extensive optimization.

REFERENCES

1. Woolf AD, Pfleger B. Burden of major musculoskeletal conditions. *Bull World Health Organ* 2003;81:646–56.
2. ASTM E. 2456-06. Standard Terminology Relating to Nanotechnology 2007.
3. Wei Q. *Functional Nanofibers and Their Applications*: Elsevier; 2012.
4. Pisignano D. *Polymer Nanofibers: Building Blocks for Nanotechnology*: RSC; 2013.
5. Nayak R, Padhye R, Kyratzis IL, Truong Y, Arnold L. Recent advances in nanofibre fabrication techniques. *Text Res J* 2012;82(2):129–47.
6. De Vrieze S, Van Camp T, Nelvig A, Hagström B, Westbroek P, De Clerck K. The effect of temperature and humidity on electrospinning. *J Mater Sci* 2009;44:1357–62.
7. Deitzel JM, Kleinmeyer J, Harris D, Tan NB. The effect of processing variables on the morphology of electrospun nanofibers and textiles. *Polymer* 2001;42:261–72.
8. Huang C, Chen S, Lai C, Reneker DH, Qiu H, Ye Y, et al. Electrospun polymer nanofibres with small diameters. *Nanotechnology* 2006;17:1558–63.
9. Samavedi S, Vaidya P, Gaddam P, Whittington AR, Goldstein AS. Electrospun meshes possessing region-wise differences in fiber orientation, diameter, chemistry and mechanical properties for engineering bone-ligament-bone tissues. *Biotechnol Bioeng* 2014;111:2549–59.
10. Vimal SK, Ahamad N, Katti DS. A simple method for fabrication of electrospun fibers with controlled degree of alignment having potential for nerve regeneration applications. *Mater Sci Eng C* 2016;63:616–27.
11. He J, Zhou Y, Wang L, Liu R, Qi K, Cui S. Fabrication of continuous nanofiber core-spun yarn by a novel electrospinning method. *Fiber Polym* 2014;15:2061–5.
12. Qu H, Wei S, Guo Z. Coaxial electrospun nanostructures and their applications. *J Mater Chem A* 2013;1:11513–28.
13. Wang YF, Guo HF, Ying DJ. Multilayer scaffold of electrospun PLA–PCL–collagen nanofibers as a dural substitute. *J Biomed Mater Res B Appl Biomater* 2013;101:1359–66.
14. Thayer PS, Dimling AF, Plessl DS, Hahn MR, Guelcher SA, Dahlgren LA, et al. Cellularized cylindrical fiber/hydrogel composites for ligament tissue engineering. *Biomacromolecules* 2013;15:75–83.
15. Bhattacharjee A, Kumar K, Arora A, Katti DS. Fabrication and characterization of Pluronic modified poly (hydroxybutyrate) fibers for potential wound dressing applications. *Mater Sci Eng C* 2016;63:266–73.
16. Padron S, Fuentes A, Caruntu D, Lozano K. Experimental study of nanofiber production through forcespinning. *J Appl Phys* 2013;113:024318.
17. Baker BM, Trappmann B, Wang WY, Sakar MS, Kim IL, Shenoy VB, et al. Cell-mediated fibre recruitment drives extracellular matrix mechanosensing in engineered fibrillar microenvironments. *Nat Mater* 2015;14:1262–68.
18. Zhang C, Yuan H, Liu H, Chen X, Lu P, Zhu T, et al. Well-aligned chitosan-based ultrafine fibers committed teno-lineage differentiation of human induced pluripotent stem cells for Achilles tendon regeneration. *Biomaterials* 2015;53:716–30.
19. Shang S, Yang F, Cheng X, Walboomers XF, Jansen JA. The effect of electrospun fibre alignment on the behaviour of rat periodontal ligament cells. *Eur Cell Mater* 2010;19:180–92.

20. Erisken C, Zhang X, Moffat KL, Levine WN, Lu HH. Scaffold fiber diameter regulates human tendon fibroblast growth and differentiation. *Tissue Eng Part A* 2012;19:519–28.
21. Cardwell RD, Dahlgren LA, Goldstein AS. Electrospun fibre diameter, not alignment, affects mesenchymal stem cell differentiation into the tendon/ligament lineage. *J Tissue Eng Regen Med* 2014;8:937–45.
22. Whited BM, Rylander MN. The influence of electrospun scaffold topography on endothelial cell morphology, alignment, and adhesion in response to fluid flow. *Biotechnol Bioeng* 2014;111:184–95.
23. Ishii H, Ishii M, Nagao D, Konno M. Advanced synthesis for monodisperse polymer nanoparticles in aqueous media with sub-millimolar surfactants. *Polymer* 2014;55:2772–79.
24. Rhee M, Valencia PM, Rodriguez MI, Langer R, Farokhzad OC, Karnik R. Synthesis of size-tunable polymeric nanoparticles enabled by 3D hydrodynamic flow focusing in single-layer microchannels. *Adv Mater* 2011;23:H79–83.
25. Sodipo BK, Aziz AA. Recent advances in synthesis and surface modification of superparamagnetic iron oxide nanoparticles with silica. *J Magn Magn Mater* 2016;416:275–91.
26. Abedini A, Bakar AAA, Larki F, Menon PS, Islam MS, Shaari S. Recent advances in shape-controlled synthesis of noble metal nanoparticles by radiolysis route. *Nanoscale Res Lett* 2016;11:1–13.
27. Sakai T, Alexandridis P. Ag and Au monometallic and bimetallic colloids: morphogenesis in amphiphilic block copolymer solutions. *Chem Mater* 2006;18:2577–83.
28. Wu W, Zhou T, Berliner A, Banerjee P, Zhou S. Smart core–shell hybrid nanogels with Ag nanoparticle core for cancer cell imaging and gel shell for pH-regulated drug delivery. *Chem Mater* 2010;22:1966–76.
29. Kumar KS, Kumar VB, Paik P. Recent advancement in functional core-shell nanoparticles of polymers: synthesis, physical properties, and applications in medical biotechnology. *J Nanopart* 2013;2013:1–24.
30. Lipski AM, Pino CJ, Haselton FR, Chen IW, Shastri VP. The effect of silica nanoparticle-modified surfaces on cell morphology, cytoskeletal organization and function. *Biomaterials* 2008;29:3836–46.
31. Nandagiri VK, Gentile P, Chiono V, Tonda-Turo C, Matsiko A, Ramtoola Z, et al. Incorporation of PLGA nanoparticles into porous chitosan–gelatin scaffolds: influence on the physical properties and cell behavior. *J Mech Behav Biomed Mater* 2011;4:1318–27.
32. Gentile P, Bellucci D, Sola A, Mattu C, Cannillo V, Ciardelli G. Composite scaffolds for controlled drug release: role of the polyurethane nanoparticles on the physical properties and cell behaviour. *J Mech Behav Biomed Mater* 2015;44:53–60.
33. Gaharwar AK, Mukundan S, Karaca E, Dolatshahi-Pirouz A, Patel A, Rangarajan K, et al. Nanoclay-enriched poly (ε-caprolactone) electrospun scaffolds for osteogenic differentiation of human mesenchymal stem cells. *Tissue Eng Part A* 2014;20:2088–101.
34. Sridhar S, Venugopal JR, Sridhar R, Ramakrishna S. Cardiogenic differentiation of mesenchymal stem cells with gold nanoparticle loaded functionalized nanofibers. *Colloids Surf B Biointerfaces* 2015;134:346–54.
35. Liu S, Tay LM, Anggara R, Chuah YJ, Kang Y. Long-term tracking mesenchymal stem cell differentiation with photostable fluorescent nanoparticles. *ACS Appl Mater Interfaces* 2016;8:11925–33.
36. Balasundaram G, Sato M, Webster TJ. Using hydroxyapatite nanoparticles and decreased crystallinity to promote osteoblast adhesion similar to functionalizing with RGD. *Biomaterials* 2006;27:2798–805.
37. Oliveira JM, Sousa RA, Kotobuki N, Tadokoro M, Hirose M, Mano JF, et al. The osteogenic differentiation of rat bone marrow stromal cells cultured with dexamethasone-loaded carboxymethylchitosan/poly(amidoamine) dendrimer nanoparticles. *Biomaterials* 2009;30:804–13.

38. Marsich E, Bellomo F, Turco G, Travan A, Donati I, Paoletti S. Nano-composite scaffolds for bone tissue engineering containing silver nanoparticles: preparation, characterization and biological properties. *J Mater Sci Mater Med* 2013;24:1799–807.

39. Andersen MO, Nygaard JV, Burns JS, Raarup MK, Nyengaard JR, Bunger C, et al. siRNA nanoparticle functionalization of nanostructured scaffolds enables controlled multilineage differentiation of stem Cells. *Mol Ther* 2010;18:2018–27.

40. Huang DM, Hsiao JK, Chen YC, Chien LY, Yao M, Chen YK, et al. The promotion of human mesenchymal stem cell proliferation by superparamagnetic iron oxide nanoparticles. *Biomaterials* 2009;30:3645–51.

41. Shang L, Nienhaus K, Nienhaus GU. Engineered nanoparticles interacting with cells: size matters. *J Nanobiotechnology* 2014;12:5.

42. Shi Z, Huang X, Cai Y, Tang R, Yang D. Size effect of hydroxyapatite nanoparticles on proliferation and apoptosis of osteoblast-like cells. *Acta Biomater* 2009;5:338–45.

43. Chen J, Hessler JA, Putchakayala K, Panama BK, Khan DP, Hong S, et al. Cationic nanoparticles induce nanoscale disruption in living cell plasma membranes. *J Phys Chem B* 2009;113:11179–85.

44. Huang X, Teng X, Chen D, Tang F, He J. The effect of the shape of mesoporous silica nanoparticles on cellular uptake and cell function. *Biomaterials* 2010;31:438–48.

45. Mitchell DT, Lee SB, Trofin L, Li N, Nevanen TK, Söderlund H, et al. Smart nanotubes for bioseparations and biocatalysis. *J Am Chem Soc* 2002;124:11864–5.

46. Baughman RH, Zakhidov AA, de Heer WA. Carbon nanotubes – the route toward applications. *Science* 2002;297:787–92.

47. Eatemadi A, Daraee H, Karimkhanloo H, Kouhi M, Zarghami N, Akbarzadeh A, et al. Carbon nanotubes: properties, synthesis, purification, and medical applications. *Nanoscale Res Lett* 2014;9:393–405.

48. Li X, Cui R, Liu W, Sun L, Yu B, Fan Y, et al. The use of nanoscaled fibers or tubes to improve biocompatibility and bioactivity of biomedical materials. *J Nanomater* 2013;2013:14–30.

49. Azadmanjiri J, Wang PY, Pingle H, Kingshott P, Wang J, Srivastava VK, et al. Enhanced attachment of human mesenchymal stem cells on nanograined titania surfaces. *RSC Adv* 2016;6:55825–33.

50. Mijangos C, Hernández R, Martín J. A review on the progress of polymer nanostructures with modulated morphologies and properties, using nanoporous AAO templates. *Prog Polym Sci* 2016;54:148–82.

51. Byun J, Lee JI, Kwon S, Jeon G, Kim JK. Highly ordered nanoporous alumina on conducting substrates with adhesion enhanced by surface modification: universal templates for ultrahigh-density arrays of nanorods. *Adv Mater* 2010;22:2028–32.

52. Li S, Mark S, Kricka L. Polymeric nanotubes and nanorods for biomedical applications. *Curr Nanosci* 2009;5:182–8.

53. Chapman R, Jolliffe KA, Perrier S. Modular design for the controlled production of polymeric nanotubes from polymer/peptide conjugates. *Polym Chem* 2011;2:1956–63.

54. Brammer KS, Oh S, Gallagher JO, Jin S. Enhanced cellular mobility guided by TiO_2 nanotube surfaces. *Nano Lett* 2008;8:786–93.

55. Robinson D, Karnik S, Mills DK. Stem cell proliferation and differentiation through capped clay nanotubes. 32nd Southern Biomedical Engineering Conference (SBEC) 2016; IEEE; 25–6.

56. Namgung S, Baik KY, Park J, Hong S. Controlling the growth and differentiation of human mesenchymal stem cells by the arrangement of individual carbon nanotubes. *ACS Nano* 2011;5:7383–90.

57. Park J, Bauer S, Schlegel KA, Neukam FW, von der Mark K, Schmuki P. TiO_2 nanotube surfaces: 15 nm – an optimal length scale of surface topography for cell adhesion and differentiation. *Small* 2009;5:666–71.

58. Lv L, Liu Y, Zhang P, Zhang X, Liu J, Chen T, et al. The nanoscale geometry of TiO_2 nanotubes influences the osteogenic differentiation of human adipose-derived stem cells by modulating H3K4 trimethylation. *Biomaterials* 2015;39:193–205.

59. Kim HN, Jiao A, Hwang NS, Kim MS, Kim DH, Suh KY. Nanotopography-guided tissue engineering and regenerative medicine. *Adv Drug Deliv Rev* 2013;65:536–58.

60. Qian T, Wang Y. Micro/nano-fabrication technologies for cell biology. *Med Biol Eng Comput* 2010;48:1023–32.

61. Chung K, Dequach JA, Christman KL. Nanopatterned interfaces for controlling cell behavior. *Nano Life* 2010;1:63–77.

62. Salaita K, Wang Y, Mirkin CA. Applications of dip-pen nanolithography. *Nat Nanotechnol* 2007;2:145–55.

63. Kim DH, Provenzano PP, Smith CL, Levchenko A. Matrix nanotopography as a regulator of cell function. *J Cell Biol* 2012;197:351–60.

64. Kim J, Kim HN, Lim KT, Kim Y, Seonwoo H, Park SH, et al. Designing nanotopographical density of extracellular matrix for controlled morphology and function of human mesenchymal stem cells. *Sci Rep* 2013;3:3552.

65. Wang X, Li S, Yan C, Liu P, Ding J. Fabrication of RGD micro/nanopattern and corresponding study of stem cell differentiation. *Nano Lett* 2015;15:1457–67.

66. Padmanabhan J, Kinser ER, Stalter MA, Duncan-Lewis C, Balestrini JL, Sawyer AJ, et al. Engineering cellular response using nanopatterned bulk metallic glass. *ACS Nano* 2014;8:4366–75.

67. Wang X, Ye K, Li Z, Yan C, Ding J. Adhesion, proliferation, and differentiation of mesenchymal stem cells on RGD nanopatterns of varied nanospacings. *Organogenesis* 2013;9:280–6.

68. Wang X, Yan C, Ye K, He Y, Li Z, Ding J. Effect of RGD nanospacing on differentiation of stem cells. *Biomaterials* 2013;34:2865–74.

69. Downing TL, Soto J, Morez C, Houssin T, Fritz A, Yuan F, et al. Biophysical regulation of epigenetic state and cell reprogramming. *Nat Mater* 2013;12:1154–62.

70. Camargo PHC, Satyanarayana KG, Wypych F. Nanocomposites: synthesis, structure, properties and new application opportunities. *Mater Res* 2009;12:1–39.

71. Liu H. *Nanocomposites for Musculoskeletal Tissue Regeneration*: Woodhead Publishing USA; 2016.

72. Gu BK, Choi DJ, Park SJ, Kim MS, Kang CM, Kim C-H. 3-Dimensional bioprinting for tissue engineering applications. *Biomater Res* 2016;20:1.

73. Lee JH, Shin YC, Lee S-M, Jin OS, Kang SH, Hong SW, et al. Enhanced osteogenesis by reduced graphene oxide/hydroxyapatite nanocomposites. *Sci Rep* 2015;5:18833.

74. Barlas F, Seleci DA, Ozkan M, Demir B, Seleci M, Aydin M, et al. Folic acid modified clay/polymer nanocomposites for selective cell adhesion. *J Mater Chem B* 2014;2:6412–21.

75. Kumar A, Young C, Farina J, Witzl A, Marks ED. Novel nanocomposite biomaterial to differentiate bone marrow mesenchymal stem cells to the osteogenic lineage for bone restoration. *J Orthop Translat* 2015;3:105–13.

76. He Y, Dong Y, Cui F, Chen X, Lin R. Ectopic osteogenesis and scaffold biodegradation of nano-hydroxyapatite-chitosan in a rat model. *PLoS One* 2015;10:e0135366.

77. D'Angelo F, Armentano I, Cacciotti I, Tiribuzi R, Quattrocelli M, Del Gaudio C, et al. Tuning multi/pluri-potent stem cell fate by electrospun poly (L-lactic acid)-calcium-deficient hydroxyapatite nanocomposite mats. *Biomacromolecules* 2012;13:1350–60.

78. Seda Kehr N, Riehemann K. Controlled cell growth and cell migration in periodic mesoporous organosilica/alginate nanocomposite hydrogels. *Adv Healthcare Mater* 2016;5:193–7.

79. Bhowmick A, Mitra T, Gnanamani A, Das M, Kundu PP. Development of biomimetic nanocomposites as bone extracellular matrix for human osteoblastic cells. *Carbohyd Polym* 2016;141:82–91.

80. Gong T, Xie J, Liao J, Zhang T, Lin S, Lin Y. Nanomaterials and bone regeneration. *Bone Res* 2015;3:15029.

81. Liu X, Jin X, Ma PX. Nanofibrous hollow microspheres self-assembled from star-shaped polymers as injectable cell carriers for knee repair. *Nat Mater* 2011;10:398–406.

82. Wu YN, Law JBK, He AY, Low HY, Hui JH, Lim CT, et al. Substrate topography determines the fate of chondrogenesis from human mesenchymal stem cells resulting in specific cartilage phenotype formation. *Nanomedicine* 2014;10:1507–16.

83. Chahine NO, Collette NM, Thomas CB, Genetos DC, Loots GG. Nanocomposite scaffold for chondrocyte growth and cartilage tissue engineering: effects of carbon nanotube surface functionalization. *Tissue Eng Part A* 2014;20:2305–15.

84. Shi D, Xu X, Ye Y, Song K, Cheng Y, Di J, et al. Photo-cross-linked scaffold with kartogenin-encapsulated nanoparticles for cartilage regeneration. *ACS Nano* 2016;10:1292–9.

85. Rezvani Z, Venugopal J, Urbanska A, Mills D, Ramakrishna S, Mozafari M. A bird's eye view on the use of electrospun nanofibrous scaffolds for bone tissue engineering: current state-of-the-art, emerging directions and future trends. *Nanomedicine* 2016;12(7):2181–200.

86. Frohbergh ME, Katsman A, Botta GP, Lazarovici P, Schauer CL, Wegst UG, et al. Electrospun hydroxyapatite-containing chitosan nanofibers crosslinked with genipin for bone tissue engineering. *Biomaterials* 2012;33:9167–78.

87. Ruckh TT, Kumar K, Kipper MJ, Popat KC. Osteogenic differentiation of bone marrow stromal cells on poly (ε-caprolactone) nanofiber scaffolds. *Acta Biomater* 2010;6:2949–59.

88. Zhang H, Fu QW, Sun TW, Chen F, Qi C, Wu J, et al. Amorphous calcium phosphate, hydroxyapatite and poly (D, L-lactic acid) composite nanofibers: electrospinning preparation, mineralization and in vivo bone defect repair. *Colloids Surf B: Biointerfaces* 2015;136:27–36.

89. Chahal S, Hussain FSJ, Kumar A, Yusoff MM, Rasad MSBA. Electrospun hydroxyethyl cellulose nanofibers functionalized with calcium phosphate coating for bone tissue engineering. *RSC Adv* 2015;5:29497–504.

90. Kwak S, Haider A, Gupta KC, Kim S, Kang IK. Micro/nano multilayered scaffolds of PLGA and collagen by alternately electrospinning for bone tissue engineering. *Nanoscale Res Lett* 2016;11:1–16.

91. Wang J, Cui X, Zhou Y, Xiang Q. Core-shell PLGA/collagen nanofibers loaded with recombinant FN/CDHs as bone tissue engineering scaffolds. *Connect Tissue Res* 2014;55:292–8.

92. Cattalini J, Hoppe A, Pishbin F, Roether J, Boccaccini A, Lucangioli S, et al. Novel nanocomposite biomaterials with controlled copper/calcium release capability for bone tissue engineering multifunctional scaffolds. *J R Soc Interface* 2015;12:20150509.

93. Wang Q, Gu Z, Jamal S, Detamore MS, Berkland C. Hybrid hydroxyapatite nanoparticle colloidal gels are injectable fillers for bone tissue engineering. *Tissue Eng Part A* 2013;19:2586–93.

94. Heo DN, Ko WK, Bae MS, Lee JB, Lee DW, Byun W, et al. Enhanced bone regeneration with a gold nanoparticle–hydrogel complex. *J Mater Chem B* 2014;2:1584–93.

95. Young PS, Tsimbouri PM, Gadegaard N, Meek RM, Dalby MJ. Osteoclastogenesis/osteoblastogenesis using human bone marrow-derived cocultures on nanotopographical polymer surfaces. *Nanomedicine* 2015;10:949–57.

96. Kim J, Bae WG, Lim KT, Jang KJ, Oh S, Jang KJ, et al. Density of nanopatterned surfaces for designing bone tissue engineering scaffolds. *Mater Lett* 2014;130:227–31.

97. Li X, Liu H, Niu X, Yu B, Fan Y, Feng Q, et al. The use of carbon nanotubes to induce osteogenic differentiation of human adipose-derived MSCs in vitro and ectopic bone formation in vivo. *Biomaterials* 2012;33:4818–27.

98. Barrientos-Durán A, Carpenter EM, Zur Nieden NI, Malinin TI, Rodríguez-Manzaneque JC, Zanello LP. Carboxyl-modified single-wall carbon nanotubes improve bone tissue formation in vitro and repair in an in vivo rat model. *Int J Nanomed.* 2014;9:4277.

99. Shearn JT, Kinneberg KR, Dyment NA, Galloway MT, Kenter K, Wylie C, et al. Tendon tissue engineering: progress, challenges, and translation to the clinic. *J Musculoskelet Neuronal Interact* 2011;11:163.

100. Nau T, Teuschl A. Regeneration of the anterior cruciate ligament: current strategies in tissue engineering. *World J Orthop* 2015;6:127.

101. Wu HY, Zhang F, Yue XX, Ming JF, Zuo BQ. Wet-spun silk fibroin scaffold with hierarchical structure for ligament tissue engineering. *Mater Lett* 2014;135:63–6.

102. Naghashzargar E, Farè S, Catto V, Bertoldi S, Semnani D, Karbasi S, et al. Nano/micro hybrid scaffold of PCL or P3HB nanofibers combined with silk fibroin for tendon and ligament tissue engineering. *J Appl Biomater Funct Mater* 2015;13(2):156–68.

103. Pauly HM, Kelly DJ, Popat KC, Trujillo NA, Dunne NJ, McCarthy HO, et al. Mechanical properties and cellular response of novel electrospun nanofibers for ligament tissue engineering: effects of orientation and geometry. *J Mech Behav Biomed Mater* 2016;61:258–70.

104. Mathew AP, Oksman K, Pierron D, Harmand MF. Biocompatible fibrous networks of cellulose nanofibres and collagen crosslinked using genipin: potential as artificial ligament/tendons. *Macromol Biosci* 2013;13:289–98.

105. Sheikh FA, Macossay J, Cantu T, Zhang X, Hassan MS, Salinas ME, et al. Imaging, spectroscopy, mechanical, alignment and biocompatibility studies of electrospun medical grade polyurethane (Carbothane™ 3575A) nanofibers and composite nanofibers containing multiwalled carbon nanotubes. *J Mech Behav Biomed Mater* 2015;41:189–98.

106. Empson YM, Ekwueme EC, Hong JK, Paynter DM, Kwansa AL, Brown C, et al. High elastic modulus nanoparticles: a novel tool for subfailure connective tissue matrix damage. *Transl Res* 2014;164:244–57.

107. Iannone M, Ventre M, Formisano L, Casalino L, Patriarca EJ, Netti PA. Nanoengineered surfaces for focal adhesion guidance trigger mesenchymal stem cell self-organization and tenogenesis. *Nano Lett* 2015;15:1517–25.

108. Chung EJ, Sugimoto MJ, Koh JL, Ameer GA. A biodegradable tri-component graft for anterior cruciate ligament reconstruction. *J Tissue Eng Regen Med* DOI:10.1002/term.1966.

109. Chen MC, Sun YC, Chen YH. Electrically conductive nanofibers with highly oriented structures and their potential application in skeletal muscle tissue engineering. *Acta Biomater* 2013;9:5562–72.

110. Choi JS, Lee SJ, Christ GJ, Atala A, Yoo JJ. The influence of electrospun aligned poly (epsilon-caprolactone)/collagen nanofiber meshes on the formation of self-aligned skeletal muscle myotubes. *Biomaterials* 2008;29:2899–906.

111. Cooper A, Jana S, Bhattarai N, Zhang M. Aligned chitosan-based nanofibers for enhanced myogenesis. *J Mater Chem* 2010;20:8904–11.

112. Ku SH, Lee SH, Park CB. Synergic effects of nanofiber alignment and electroactivity on myoblast differentiation. *Biomaterials* 2012;33:6098–104.

113. Aviss K, Gough J, Downes S. Aligned electrospun polymer fibres for skeletal muscle regeneration. *Eur Cell Mater* 2010;19:193–204.

114. Fraczek-Szczypta A, Menaszek E, Blazewicz S, Adu J, Shevchenko R, Syeda TB, et al. Influence of different types of carbon nanotubes on muscle cell response. *Mater Sci Eng C* 2015;46:218–25.

115. Zhao C, Andersen H, Ozyilmaz B, Ramaprabhu S, Pastorin G, Ho HK. Spontaneous and specific myogenic differentiation of human mesenchymal stem cells on polyethylene glycol-linked multi-walled carbon nanotube films for skeletal muscle engineering. *Nanoscale* 2015;7:18239–49.

116. Krueger E, Chang AN, Brown D, Eixenberger J, Brown R, Rastegar S, et al. Graphene foam as a 3-dimensional platform for myotube growth. *ACS Biomater Sci Eng* 2016;2.8:1234–41.

117. Barua S, Gogoi B, Aidew L, Buragohain AK, Chattopadhyay P, Karak N. Sustainable resource based hyperbranched epoxy nanocomposite as an infection resistant, biodegradable, implantable muscle scaffold. *ACS Sustainable Chem Eng* 2015;3:1136–44.

118. Mooney E, Mackle JN, Blond DJ-P, O'Cearbhaill E, Shaw G, Blau WJ, et al. The electrical stimulation of carbon nanotubes to provide a cardiomimetic cue to MSCs. *Biomaterials* 2012;33:6132–9.

119. Chen Z, Wang P, Wei B, Mo X, Cui F. Electrospun collagen–chitosan nanofiber: a biomimetic extracellular matrix for endothelial cell and smooth muscle cell. *Acta Biomater* 2010;6:372–82.

120. Dvir T, Bauer M, Schroeder A, Tsui JH, Anderson DG, Langer R, et al. Nanoparticles targeting the infarcted heart. *Nano Lett* 2011;11:4411–4.

121. Kim J, Cao L, Shvartsman D, Silva EA, Mooney DJ. Targeted delivery of nanoparticles to ischemic muscle for imaging and therapeutic angiogenesis. *Nano Lett* 2010;11:694–700.

CHAPTER 7

3D Bioprinting for Regenerative Engineering

Nathan J. Castro, Wei Zhu, Haitao Cui,

Se-Jun Lee, and Lijie Grace Zhang

The George Washington University

CONTENTS

7.1 INTRODUCTION

Tissue engineering (TE) holds great promise for developing methods for repairing tissue damage, thus preventing the need for more invasive procedures. TE applies the principles of engineering and life sciences for the development of biological substitutes to restore, maintain, or improve tissue function [1]. For orthopedic, neural, and vascular tissue regeneration, autologous stem cells can be harvested from the patient, expanded *in vitro*, and subsequently cultivated using a three-dimensional (3D) scaffold. After cultivation, the scaffold can effectively be transplanted into the patient after cell differentiation for enhanced tissue integration [2–9]. Conventional scaffold fabrication techniques, such as particle leaching [10–12] and gas foaming [13–16], have been used to manufacture porous scaffolding for tissue regeneration. Although they have been shown to be effective *in vitro*, limitations exist with regard to insufficient pore interconnectivity, leading to poor tissue integration where host tissue integration is imperative to long-term success. 3D bioprinting technologies have garnered greater attention for the fabrication of highly ordered tissue engineered scaffolds. The scope of this chapter will serve to present various 3D bioprinting modalities and nanobiomaterials for osteochondral, neural, and vascular tissue regeneration. In addition, discussions on the current challenges inhibiting efficient and long-term efficacy of said scaffolds are included.

7.2 3D PRINTING TECHNIQUES

Rapid prototyping or 3D printing is an enabling technology whose main attribute is to reduce product development and manufacturing times, as well as cost, resulting in an increase in market competitiveness [17]. Although this definition focuses on manufacturing, the fundamental ideas presented hold true for TE applications of 3D printing or as we shall refer to 3D printing in the context of bioactive scaffold fabrication as "bioprinting." 3D bioprinting can readily enable scientists and doctors to efficiently engineer personalized scaffolds for patient-specific treatment. In addition, patients will not have to wait for a viable donor, surrender to total joint replacement, or endure the loss of limb functionality at an early age due to disease progression, but they will instead be treated with cell-laden or bioactive 3D scaffolds. Advances in biomaterials research is a critical component to the realization of functional and efficient scaffolding where processability and biocompatibility must be considered. Several technologies for 3D bioactive scaffold fabrication exist to include: stereolithography (SL), fused deposition modeling (FDM), selective laser sintering (SLS), extrusion, and inkjet bioprinting, as shown in Figure 7.1. In the following sections, we will discuss each technology in depth as they relate to TE scaffold fabrication.

7.2.1 Stereolithography

As one of the oldest rapid prototyping technologies, SL can be readily employed to manufacture stratified, multilayered scaffolds through ultraviolet-visible photopolymerization of photocurable resins; examples of SL setup and printed scaffolds are shown in Figure 7.2. The geometry and architecture of the cured resin can be readily controlled by a focused laser beam (beam scanning) [19–24] or digital masks projected from computer-aided design interfaces (mask-image-projection) [25–28]. This technology remains one of the most powerful and versatile, exhibiting the highest fabrication accuracy. It is largely a bottom-up process although research does exist on top-down fabrication methods.

Some challenges associated with SL include available biomaterials, material toxicity complications due to incorporated photoinitiators, and inadequate cell adhesion. Although the breadth of materials is steadily increasing, the resultant mechanical properties of fabricated scaffolds are equally broad, but still lack the toughness required for load-bearing orthopedic applications. Additionally, for implantation, a compounding complication is the presence of photoinitiators which are added to the liquid resin to expedite cross-linking [29]. These materials must be carefully controlled and monitored to ensure that

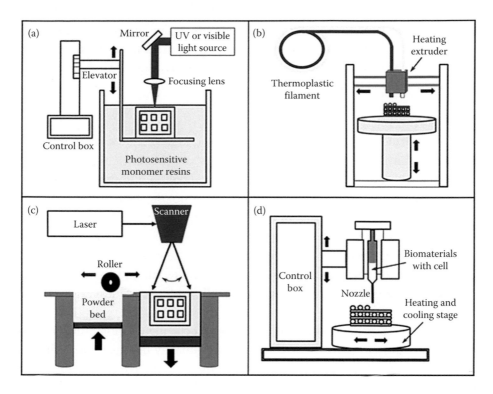

FIGURE 7.1 Schematics of 3D bioprinting techniques discussed: (a) stereolithography (mask image-projection), (b) fused deposition modeling, (c) selective laser sintering, and (d) extrusion or inkjet bioprinting. Modified and reproduced with permission from Gu et al. [18].

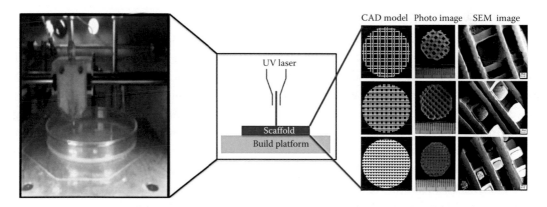

FIGURE 7.2 Images of an SL printer (beam-scanning model) and resultant scaffolds as well as a schematic of the process (center). Adapted from Castro et al. [30].

in vivo degradation is not marred with excessive buildup, leading to cytotoxicity, inadequate tissue integration, and resultant failure. Scaffolds fabricated by SL are largely based on poly(ethylene glycol) hydrogels which are intrinsically non-cell adherent. Often, micro-/nanoparticles, growth factors, or binding proteins must be incorporated to improve cellular attachment and overall tissue formation. In order for this technology to progress toward clinically relevant tissue engineered scaffolds, more research on biocompatible materials is needed. Photocross-linkable natural polymers, such as gelatin methacrylate, hyaluronic acid (HA) methacrylate, and others, are an emerging research area in this field which may address some of these challenges.

7.2.2 Fused Deposition Modeling

FDM is the most widely used 3D printing technique due to financial accessibility, ease of use, and quick printing time. This technique utilizes thermoplastic filaments, which are heated to their melting point or a semi-molten state, allowing it to flow and subsequently solidify upon the printing stage through an extrusion nozzle without the need for additional cross-linking agents or processes [31, 32]. Due to this process, the material choices for FDM are limited, as raw materials need to be processed into a rigid filament [33]. The resolution of FDM printed constructs is relatively low, which is directly governed by the nozzle diameter, rheological properties of the material, and the distance between the substrate and the nozzle, resulting in an overall resolution of several hundredths of micrometers.

Compared to the 3D printed hydrogel-based constructs, FDM bioprinting is a relatively well-explored modality in hard tissue engineering primarily because several biomaterial filaments with high mechanical strength are currently commercially available, including poly(lactic acid) (PLA), poly(ε-caprolactone) (PCL), poly(vinyl alcohol), and others [34, 35]. Moreover, the open source nature of many affordable FDM printers ensures frequent development and improvements for multiple materials and other technologies, leading to the availability of more biocompatible filaments [33].

7.2.3 Selective Laser Sintering

For the manufacture of hard tissue and rigid support structures, SLS is a suitable technique for the manufacture of orthopedic tissue scaffolds. This process uses a focused laser similar to SL to fuse nano-/microparticles/powders together into a solid component, as shown in Figure 7.3. This technique can also be used with composite slurries and combinations of powdered particles and gels in a similar manner. Both techniques involve the spreading of a thin layer of powder/slurry, exposure of deposited layer with a high-power laser for fusion/solidification, and repeating as necessary to obtain the predesigned 3D structure [36–41]. Solidification of the slurry is achieved through evaporation of the liquid phase which allows for fusion of the solid phase material. The process of bonding/fusing creates surfaces with favorable roughness at scales desirable for cell adhesion.

Benefits of this technique include the ability to integrate the Food and Drug Administration (FDA)-approved materials for orthopedic implantation. In addition, research exists on SLS of pure and alloyed titanium (Ti) powder with silica sol, cobalt chrome (CoCr), and Ti6Al4V alloys in a biphasic system consisting of bioactive hydroxyapatite and silica sol [43, 44]. These studies illustrated successful fabrication and evaluation of SLS-based components constructed with materials previously approved as safe for implantation. This technology holds promise for constructing smaller, individualized components for implantation as a preventative measure before larger, more invasive procedures

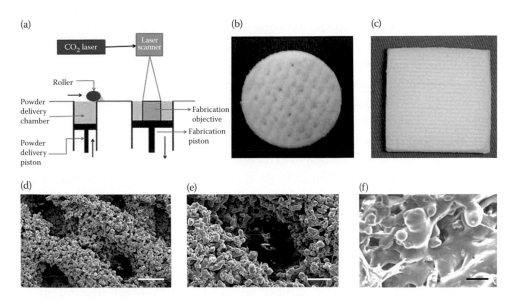

FIGURE 7.3 Schematic of SLS system (a) and images of printed scaffolds (b–c). Scanning electron micrographs of SLS printed scaffolds (d–f). Scale bars = 500 μm (d), 200 μm (e), and 100 μm (f). Modified and reprinted with permission from Liao et al. [42].

or full joint replacement are warranted. Further evolution of this technique can lead to efficient and viable scaffolds for bone and other hard tissues by facilitating clinical approval and increasing integration based on the extensive use of FDA-approved materials, which is a considerable benefit not shared by most other bioprinting techniques at the present time.

Some drawbacks of SLS printing are largely predicated on equipment cost; SLS-based printers are considerably more expensive compared to other 3D printing technologies. Proper manufacturing of components is a careful balance between laser strength, speed, and spacing to achieve desired scaffold bulk properties. Similar to other 3D bioprinting techniques, SLS processing parameters and inherent material properties of powders have significant implications on the overall performance of the sintered construct [45].

7.2.4 Extrusion Bioprinting

Extrusion bioprinting is an additive manufacturing technique for the fabrication of 3D tissue engineered scaffolds where cell-laden and/or non-cell-laden materials are extruded as a viscous fluid through a syringe into tubes or spheroids and cured using ultraviolet radiation, chemical cross-linking agents, or time-dependent solidification [46]. Extrusion bioprinting allows for the use of one or multiple syringes containing discrete cell types or bioactive materials leading to the formation of more compositionally complex constructs. This capability allows for the integration of cells and biomaterials to replicate physiologically relevant spatial orientation, geometries, and complexities [47]. The main caveat of this technology is in the necessity for high-viscosity bioprinting materials providing adequate surface tension to self-support or to be submerged in a liquid media of matching density to provide support while cross-linking [48].

The ability to directly impregnate biomaterials with cells while bioprinting is certainly an advantage of these systems, thus reducing material processing. However, the bioprinted scaffolds commonly exhibit a very smooth surface, which is attributed to the extrusion and curing process. Surface morphology has extensively been linked to cell adhesion and proliferation [49, 50]. As such, additional scaffold surface modification is often necessary to create surface roughness to improve cell adhesion [51]. Furthermore, the materials currently available for syringe-based extrusion often do not possess mechanical properties suitable for implantation [46]. Although extrusion bioprinting shows promise for the rapid fabrication of cell impregnated biomaterials, more focused research is necessary for the development of extrudable, biocompatible materials possessing favorable mechanical and physical properties.

7.2.5 Inkjet Bioprinting

Inkjet bioprinting is a method of depositing bioinks containing cells and/or biological materials through the extension of commercial inkjet printers. Much like the preceding extrusion technology, inkjet bioprinting is a bottom-up scaffold fabrication technique in which cells and hydrogels can be directly and precisely printed into 3D tissue-engineered scaffolds, as illustrated in Figure 7.4. Compared to "filament"-based extrusion bioprinting, inkjet bioprinting relies on various energy sources (thermal-, electric-, laser beam-, acoustic-, or pneumatic-mechanisms) to pattern the bioink droplets in a high-throughput manner. Additionally, inkjet printers containing multiple print cartridges have a similar capability of allowing simultaneous printing of multiple cell types [52]. Owing to the relative accessibility and availability of commercial printers, very precise, noncontact deposition of cells can be directly applied on predesigned scaffolds.

The biggest challenge with inkjet bioprinting devices is cell settling and aggregation at the printer nozzle within the printer cartridge, which can lead to obstruction and non-uniform distribution during material deposition. Some solutions have been evaluated in an attempt to resolve this problem, such as agitation of the medium contained in the cartridge which can directly impact cell viability [54]. More research is needed to find a stand-alone material capable of acting as the cell-carrying medium within the cartridges and solidifying to a self-supporting, biocompatible scaffold on deposition.

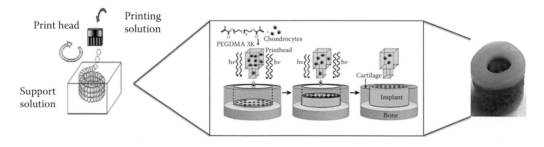

FIGURE 7.4 Schematic of inkjet bioprinting system, scaffold production schematic, and image of final scaffold created using inkjet bioprinting. Adapted and reprinted with permission from Wust et al. [53].

Some emerging research has focused on hybrid bioprinting techniques using multiple bioprinting materials wherein one contains a cell suspension and the other serves to deposit the printing substrate or "biopaper." One source acts as the cross-linking agent after contact to drive material solidification. This technique has shown positive results *in vitro* and *in vivo*, illustrating normal proliferation rates and good cell viability. Deposited cells survived and matured into functional tissue showing adequate *de novo* tissue formation [52]. This type of success is driving more advanced research and *in vivo* studies using hybrid devices, moving focus away from directly bioprinting cell-laden materials. Further research in bioink development, especially regarding direct bioprinting, could lead to continued advancement in cell printing for tissue engineering [54].

In the following sections, we will discuss three focus areas in which bioprinting has helped to advance the state of current research as well as present the benefits and current limitations as they relate to 3D bioprinting of complex tissues (osteochondral interface), vascularized tissue, and neural tissue regeneration.

7.3 3D BIOPRINTING FOR COMPLEX TISSUE REGENERATION

7.3.1 3D Bioprinting Osteochondral Tissue

Clinically, osteoarthritis (OA) is the gradual degeneration of cartilage within articulating joints, which manifests symptomatically as joint pain, impinged movement, and overall dysfunction [55]. In 2005, 47.8 million Americans were diagnosed with OA with updated projections growing to 96 million by 2050 [56]. Joint degeneration is induced by chronic or acute damage to cartilaginous tissue at the joint surface. Available surgical methods are predicated on the severity and size of the defect [57], as shown in Figure 7.5, ranging from focal-sized (<2 cm² diameter) defects where no efficient treatment options exist to complete joint degeneration requiring highly invasive complete joint arthroplasty. Less invasive methods to modulate disease progression exist, but are ineffective in recapitulating the native extracellular matrix (ECM) niche. This mismatch leads to increased defect severity and, in most severe cases, to total joint replacement. Currently, large defect tissue repair is conducted using autografts or allografts when available and feasible, but they have inherent limitations with regard to graft thickness inconsistencies [58], donor tissue harvest site [59], and graft incongruency [60]. If the damage is too severe and the supply of healthy tissue is not available for a sufficient auto- or allograft, total joint replacement is necessary to mobilize the patient.

Osteochondral tissue, at the bone-cartilage interface, is complex and includes various chemical gradients, morphological gradients, and disparate mechanical properties. Interfacial tissue engineering (ITE) is an approach that addresses the complex bi- or multiphasic nature of tissue defects where two or more disparate tissues are proximally located [61]. The basic premise relies on the introduction or elicitation of cells to the defect site by means of an appropriate scaffold, resulting in directed spatial and temporal tissue remodeling [62, 63].

To address the complex nature of osteochondral tissue, advances in scaffold design have also included biochemical cues that mimic those found within articular cartilage and subchondral bone exhibiting improved cell adhesion, proliferation, directed

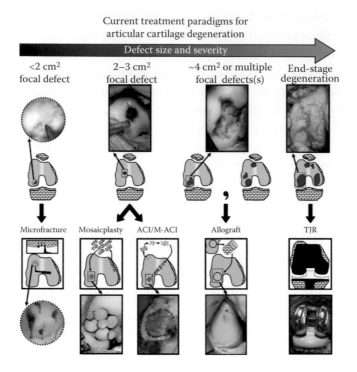

FIGURE 7.5 Current clinical treatment options for articular joint damage. Adapted and reprinted with permission from Williams et al. [57].

differentiation, and phenotypic expression [64, 65]. In addition to scaffold design, biomaterial limitations of traditional TE approaches with respect to spatial and temporal control of tissue formation and the mechanical properties of single tissue-specific constructs have proven challenging. Therefore, applying nanobiomaterials and advanced 3D bioprinting to manufacture novel biomimetic osteochondral constructs linking two distinct tissues within certain biological and mechanical constraints merits considerable focused attention.

As an emerging manufacturing technique, 3D bioprinting offers tremendous precision and control over the microarchitecture, shape, and composition of tissue scaffolds. Therefore, it greatly facilitates the development of multiphasic, predesigned microarchitectural scaffolds to direct specific tissue formation within a specific site like the osteochondral interface. Fedorovich et al. simultaneously printed osteogenic progenitor cells and chondrocytes into an intricate alginate hydrogel scaffold using bioplotting [66]. The *in vitro* and *in vivo* results showed that distinctive ECM regions were formed in different parts of the construct, which made the repair of osteochondral defects promising [66]. Gao et al. co-printed acrylated peptides and acrylated poly(ethylene glycol) with human bone marrow-derived mesenchymal stem cells (hMSCs) using an inkjet bioprinter [67]. The results demonstrated excellent mineral and cartilage matrix deposition, as well as significantly increased mechanical properties [67]. Our laboratory also designed and printed a series of biphasic 3D geometric models, using FDM printing which mimics the osteochondral region of articulate joints. The results showed that 3D printed biphasic

PLA scaffolds can promote specific stem cell differentiation and improve mechanical strength as well as interfacial integration [35].

Moreover, through the combination of bioactive factors, nanomaterials, fibers, and others, the constructs can closely mimic the native 3D extracellular environment with hierarchical nanoroughness, microstructure, and spatiotemporal bioactive cues [33, 68]. Recently, our group developed a novel nano-ink to fabricate porous and highly interconnected osteochondral scaffold with hierarchical nano-to-micro structure and spatiotemporal bioactive factor gradients using SL printing. The nano-ink combines osteo-inductive nanocrystalline hydroxyapatite and core-shell poly(lactic-co-glycolic) acid (PLGA) nanospheres encapsulated with chondrogenic transforming growth factor β1(TGF-β1). Our results showed that hMSC adhesion, proliferation, and osteochondral differentiation were greatly improved in the biomimetic graded 3D printed osteochondral construct *in vitro* [69]. In addition, Zhang et al. fabricated biphasic osteochondral composite scaffolds composed of polyethylene glycol hydrogel and β-tricalcium phosphate ceramic using SL printing technology, and subsequently implanted the scaffolds in a critical-sized rabbit trochlea defect model [70]. The animal study results showed that hyaline-like cartilage formed, along with white smooth surface and invisible margin at 24 weeks postoperatively, and that typical tidemark formed at 52 weeks. The repaired subchondral bone formed from 16 to 52 weeks in a "flow-like" gradual manner from the surrounding bone to the defect center [70]. The multilayered 3D construct containing hMSCs within a hydrogel comprised of atelocollagen and supramolecular HA was printed using an extrusion printer with multiple printing heads [71]. These printing heads ejected thermally molten PCL and liquid atelocollagen/hMSCs/bone morphogenetic protein 2 (BMP-2), Cucurbit[6]uril (CB[6])-HA/hMSCs/TGF-β, and 1,6-diaminohexane-HA to form the 3D bioactive supramolecular hydrogels for regeneration of osteochondral defects. The printed construct showed outstanding regenerative ability for the reconstruction of an osteochondral tissue in a similar rabbit knee defect model [71].

7.3.2 3D Bioprinting Vascularized Tissue

As highlighted above, multi-material bioactive scaffolds can be readily manufactured from biocompatible and bioactive materials. Although much progress has been made, several limitations persist with regard to neovascularization. Under certain constraints, cells have the capability of anastomosing to the native vasculature of the host, but due to capillary diffusion limitations, the supply of oxygen and nutrition to the cells is confined to an area of 100–200 μm [72]. Therefore, blood vessels are required for engineered tissues post implantation to overcome diffusion limitations [73]. With the exception of a few avascular tissues, i.e., cartilage, skin, and cornea, where cells can remain viable from blood vessels residing a relative distance away, vascularization is essential for most other tissues and implanted scaffolds to guarantee scaffold integration and tissue regeneration. It is known that new blood vessels will spontaneously form within transplants by invasion of host blood vessels after implantation *in vivo*, which is a result of the inflammatory wound healing process as well as the release of angiogenic factors regulated by hypoxia [73]. However, this process is slow and partial to near-complete vascularization takes weeks, resulting in localized nutrient deficiency and hypoxia within the interior of the implant. Therefore, to create more viably functional tissues, additional strategies have been developed and used in combination with 3D bioprinting for improved vascularization. Currently, several strategies are being investigated to enhance neovascularization, which includes enhanced scaffold geometry that promotes neovascularization, inclusion of angiogenic factors, and pre-vascularization of 3D printed scaffolds. In the following section, we will delve into the use of 3D bioprinting as a technology to manufacture and facilitate the formation of vascularized tissues.

The micostructural design of scaffolds is critical for *in vivo* vascularization. Studies have shown that larger pore sizes and higher interconnectivity of the scaffolds can significantly promote the growth and integrity of blood vessels [74]. Conventional scaffold manufacturing techniques, as previously mentioned, cannot be used to fabricate the complex hierarchical structure(s) necessary for vascularization. The emergence of 3D bioprinting offers a new strategy for fabricating scaffolds in a precise and tailored manner. In addition to the controlled architecture, 3D bioprinting allows for the precise deposition of multiple cell types, growth factors, and other ECM components. 3D bioprinting allows for the inclusion of more complexity to a predesigned scaffold, especially for large, complex, vascularized tissues which have varying cell types and multi-scale vascular channels.

A promising strategy to create vascularized tissues is printing scaffolds with interconnected channels followed by introducing endothelial cells (ECs) into the channels. The ECs could be directly seeded into the channels or introduced by perfused cell flow, resulting in the tubular structure formation along the interconnected channels [75a, 75b, 76]. In our recent study, we developed a highly innovative design of a vascularized tissue construct (Figure 7.6) with hierarchical architecture, using a dual 3D bioprinting platform that consisted of an FDM bioprinter and an SLA bioprinter [77]. Moreover, the bioactive factors such as BMP-2 and vascular endothelial growth factor peptides were regionally immobilized to promote osteogenesis and angiogenesis. Our results showed that a complex, microstructural, vascularized tissue with both well-organized vascular lumen and a rich capillary network was successfully formed in the 3D bioprinted tissue construct. In our study, a 3D bioprinted biomimetic fluid perfused vascular microstructure was integrated with biologically inspired, smart growth factor release system for the first time [32]. This integrated strategy not only proposes originally the cooperative biological signaling event as an external trigger of stimuli-responsive release system but also provides considerable potential for vascularized tissue regeneration induced by sequentially delivering multiple growth factors in spatiotemporal coordination. These advanced 3D bioprinting strategies coupled with novel printing materials and appropriate vascular designs could provide a highly innovative biomimetic solution for complex vascularized tissue regeneration.

7.3.3 3D Bioprinting for Neural Regeneration

Unlike the successes previously discussed regarding the regeneration of musculoskeletal tissue, nerve regeneration is very difficult to achieve because of the intrinsic complexity of the nervous system. Particularly, the central nervous system has a limited capacity to spontaneously regenerate axons after injury. Recently, neural tissue engineering has shown

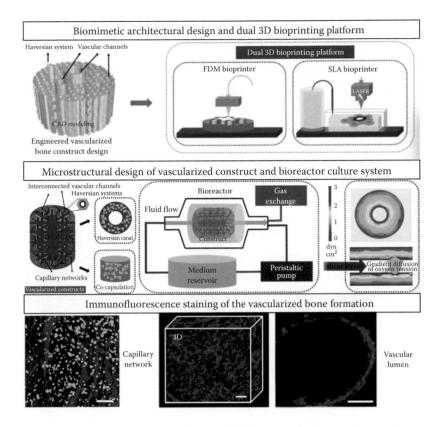

FIGURE 7.6   Novel bioprinting strategies for perfusable vascularized construct fabrication developed in our laboratory. Adapted and reprinted with permission from Cui et al. [77].

considerable promise to address currently untreatable nerve injuries and disease via the development of biomimetic 3D scaffolds. 3D scaffolds have shown to improve the development of functional network connectivity and neural synapse compared to that of 2D scaffolds [78–80]. Among many biofabrication methods, 3D bioprinting allows customized fabrication of 3D neural scaffold which possess suitable elasticity as well as organizational complexity which closely matches that of native neural tissues.

Several 3D bioprinting techniques have produced encouraging results toward the improvement of functional neural tissue [81–84]. Hsieh et al. have used customized FDM 3D printers to fabricate thermoresponsive water-based polyurethane with neural stem cells (NSCs) [84]. The results showed that injection of the NSC-laden hydrogels facilitates the repair of the damaged central nervous system (CNS) in a zebrafish embryo neural injury model. In addition, the function of an adult zebrafish with traumatic brain injury was rescued after implantation of 3D printed NSC-laden hydrogel scaffold. These findings suggested that NSCs embedded in the suitable 3D hydrogel scaffold may have the potential to improve the function of the impaired nervous system in various neurodegenerative diseases. In our recent study, we have employed SL 3D printing and co-axial electrospraying techniques to fabricate a novel 3D biomimetic neural scaffold, which has tunable porous structure, and embedded core-shell nanoparticles as a neurogenic factor delivery system [85]. Our confocal microscopy results demonstrated that scaffolds embedded with nerve growth factor (NGF) nanoparticles increased the length of neurites and directed neurite extension of PC-12 cells along the direction of fiber alignment significantly compared to that of bare hydrogel scaffold (Figure 7.7). This study shows the potential of 3D printed scaffolds with nanobiomaterials in enhancing directional growth and differentiation of neural cells.

In addition to scaffold mechanical properties, the capacity of the material to conduct electrical impulses is imperative to the overall success of neural tissue implants. Owing to the fact that neural tissue is electrically active, several studies have utilized 3D printed conductive constructs to enhance electrical stimulation of superficial and embedded cells. For example, Weng et al. have successfully used inkjet technology to print a conductive polymer composite (polypyrrole (PPy)/collagen) scaffold with incorporated electrical stimulation [86]. In this study, PPy and collagen were micro-patterned on a polyarylate film by inkjet printing for electrical stimulation within a spatially controlled system. The PPy/collagen structure enhanced PC-12 cell adherence, growth, and while under electrical stimulation, increased neurite outgrowth and orientation. In a most recent study, a mixture of graphene and PLGA polymer was utilized as a bioink for extrusion-based 3D bioprinting to create a graphene structure with a micro-resolution [87]. The resultant 3D scaffold was mechanically robust and flexible while retaining electrical conductivities. More importantly, *in vitro* experiments revealed that graphene-incorporated 3D scaffolds support hMSC adhesion, viability, proliferation, and differentiation into neuron-like cells without exposure to exogenous neurotrophic factors [87].

3D direct cell bioprinting also provides another unique opportunity to replicate the 3D spatial distribution of various cell types to mimic neural network. Recently, Tse et al. utilized a modified piezoelectric inkjet printer to print a neural cell-laden scaffold [88]. The study showed for the first time that NG108–15 neuronal cells and primary Schwann cells can be piezoelectrically printed with no adverse effects over a higher range of voltage. These results also showed that 3D bioprinted neuronal NG108 cells displayed longer neurites than those of nonprinted cells. These are only a handful of the exemplary use of 3D

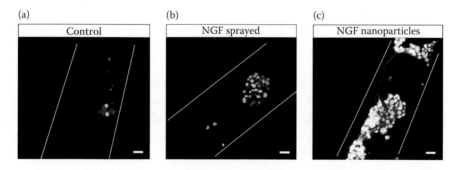

FIGURE 7.7 Confocal microscopy images of PC-12 cell growth and spreading on SL printed scaffolds after seven days of culture. (a–c) Double staining of MAP-2 and TUJ-1 to detect PC-12 differentiation on various scaffolds. Scale bar=50 µm. NGF nanoparticles represent the scaffold incorporated with NGF nanoparticles. Adapted and reprinted with permission from Lee et al. [85].

bioprinting for the replication of natural 3D cellular structures, which illustrate the usefulness of *in vitro* neural network models and functional scaffolds for various neuroscience applications.

7.3.4 New Frontier: 4D Bioprinting

3D bioprinting assumes the printed objects are static and inanimate without any state change after printing. To address this concern, 4D bioprinting emerged where the fourth dimension "time" is integrated. Different from 3D bioprinting which produces complex 3D products with fixed architecture, a programmed shape change design is involved in 4D bioprinting. 4D printed objects can alter their original shape or functionalities under an external stimulus, or the fusion and self-assembly of 4D printed cell droplets occur post printing (Figure 7.8a) [89].

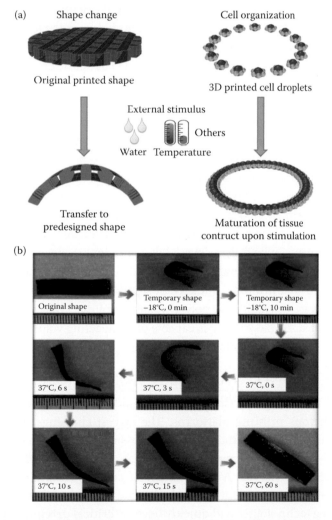

FIGURE 7.8 (a) Scheme of 4D bioprinting approaches and (b) temperature-stimulated 4D printed scaffold shape change. Adapted and reprinted with permission from Miao et al. [95].

4D bioprinting may involve the printing of smart materials which can undergo large conformational or functional changes in response to external stimuli, including temperature, water, pH, ionic strength, magnetic, or light [90, 91]. The change in the state of materials is usually reversible. Because human tissues and organs are in a body fluid environment comprising of a large amount of water and other ECM, water is one of the most popular stimuli for deforming 3D bioprinted scaffolds to fulfill a 4D bioprinting in regenerative medicine. One interesting study conducted by Gladman et al. may pave the way for water-stimulated 4D bioprinting [92]. They programmed bilayer architectures and 4D bioprinted a biomimetic hydrogel composite which can induce complex shape change after immersing in water. The hydrogel composite consisted of stiff cellulose fibrils encapsulated in a soft acrylamide matrix. By defining the elastic and swelling anisotropies through controlling the orientation of cellulose fibrils in hydrogel, the shape changes of printed construct after immersion in water can be deterministically controlled. During printing, the extruded cellulose fibrils were aligned along the nozzle movement orientation by shear force, resulting in the anisotropic stiffness of the printed filaments between the longitudinal and transverse directions. The anisotropic stiffness further induced different swelling behavior in two directions which was utilized to realize the shape change after printing.

In addition to water, temperature is another commonly used stimulus in 4D printing. Thermoresponsive shape-memory polymers have impressive shape change on temperature alteration, demonstrating an excellent candidate for temperature-stimulated 4D bioprinting. The shape memory polymers can be produced from natural or synthetic materials [93]. The thermoresponsible shape change involves a process which combines programming and recovery [94]. The programming process will deform and fix a 3D bioprinted construct into a temporary shape; on change of temperature (external stimulus), the printed construct recovers its permanent shape as initially printed. In our study, we synthesized and 4D printed a novel, renewable, natural soybean oil epoxidized acrylate [95]. The printed scaffold can be fixed a temporary shape at −18°C and then can be fully recovered to its original shape at human body temperature (37°C), indicating the considerable potential for 4D printing applications (Figure 7.8b). In addition, we found that printed scaffolds can significantly promote hMSC adhesion and proliferation in contrast to traditional polyethylene glycol diacrylate printing material. The temperature-stimulated 4D bioprinting is capable of compacting voluminous constructs into small ones and can be used for minimal invasive surgery in tissue engineering applications.

7.4 CONCLUSIONS AND FUTURE DIRECTIONS

3D bioprinting of tissue-engineered scaffolds is rapidly advancing with diverse research occurring on numerous printing platforms. The largest challenge in this field remains the ability to balance all performance objectives for successful scaffold integration within areas of biological and physical complexity, such as the osteochondral interface, highly vascularized tissues, and nerves. A large extent of current research has shown marked advancements. It should be evident through the course of this discussion that 3D (and now 4D) bioprinting technologies will quickly become critical driving forces leading to the clinical use of bioprinted scaffolds.

ACKNOWLEDGMENTS

The authors are grateful for financial support from the National Institutes of Health Director's New Innovator Award 1DP2EB020549-01, National Science Foundation Biomedical Engineering program grant #1510561, National Science Foundation Manufacturing Machines and Equipment program grant #1642186, and the March of Dimes Foundation's Gene Discovery and Translational Research Grant.

REFERENCES

1. Langer, R. and J.P. Vacanti, Tissue engineering. *Science*, 1993. 260(5110): pp. 920–926.
2. Ge, Z., et al., Histological evaluation of osteogenesis of 3D-printed poly-lactic-co-glycolic acid (PLGA) scaffolds in a rabbit model. *Biomedical Materials*, 2009. 4(2): pp. 1–7.
3. Yu, H., et al., Promotion of osteogenesis in tissue-engineered bone by pre-seeding endothelial progenitor cells-derived endothelial cells. *Journal of Orthopaedic Research*, 2008. 26(8): pp. 1147–1152.
4. Binan, L., et al., Approaches for neural tissue regeneration. *Stem Cell Reviews*, 2014. 10(1): pp. 44–59.
5. Menaa, F., A. Abdelghani, and B. Menaa, Graphene nanomaterials as biocompatible and conductive scaffolds for stem cells: impact for tissue engineering and regenerative medicine. *Journal of Tissue Engineering and Regenerative Medicine*, 2015. 9(12): pp. 1321–1338.
6. Zhu, W., et al., 3D nano/microfabrication techniques and nanobiomaterials for neural tissue regeneration. *Nanomedicine* (London), 2014. 9(6): pp. 859–875.
7. Tan, G.N., et al., Tissue engineering vascular grafts a fortiori: looking back and going forward. *Expert Opinion on Biological Therapy*, 2015. 15(2): pp. 231–244.
8. Wilhelmi, M., S. Jockenhoevel, and P. Mela, Bioartificial fabrication of regenerating blood vessel substitutes: requirements and current strategies. *Biomedizinische Technik* (Berlin), 2014. 59(3): pp. 185–195.
9. Li, S., D. Sengupta, and S. Chien, Vascular tissue engineering: from in vitro to in situ. *Wiley Interdisciplinary Reviews: Systems Biology and Medicine*, 2014. 6(1): pp. 61–76.
10. Guan, L. and J.E. Davies, Preparation and characterization of a highly macroporous biodegradable composite tissue engineering scaffold. *Journal of Biomedical Materials Research Part A*, 2004. 71(3): pp. 480–487.
11. Lebourg, M., et al., Biodegradable polycaprolactone scaffold with controlled porosity obtained by modified particle-leaching technique. *Journal of Materials Science: Materials in Medicine*, 2008. 19(5): pp. 2047–2053.
12. Wang, W., et al., In vivo restoration of full-thickness cartilage defects by poly(lactide-co-glycolide) sponges filled with fibrin gel, bone marrow mesenchymal stem cells and DNA complexes. *Biomaterials*, 2010. 31(23): pp. 5953–5965.
13. Yoo, H.S., et al., Hyaluronic acid modified biodegradable scaffolds for cartilage tissue engineering. *Biomaterials*, 2005. 26(14): pp. 1925–1933.
14. Mathieu, L.M., et al., Architecture and properties of anisotropic polymer composite scaffolds for bone tissue engineering. *Biomaterials*, 2006. 27(6): pp. 905–916.
15. Salerno, A., S. Iannace, and P.A. Netti, Graded biomimetic osteochondral scaffold prepared via CO_2 foaming and micronized NaCl leaching. *Materials Letters*, 2012. 82: pp. 137–140.
16. Prieto, E.M., et al., Injectable foams for regenerative medicine. *Wiley Interdisciplinary Reviews: Nanomedicine and Nanobiotechnology*, 2014. 6(2): pp. 136–154.
17. Pham, D.T. and R.S. Gault, A comparison of rapid prototyping technologies. *International Journal of Machine Tools & Manufacture*, 1998. 38(10–11): pp. 1257–1287.

18. Gu, B.K., et al., 3-Dimensional bioprinting for tissue engineering applications. *Biomaterials Research*, 2016. 20(1): pp. 1–8.
19. Fisher, J.P., et al., Soft and hard tissue response to photocrosslinked poly(propylene fumarate) scaffolds in a rabbit model. *Journal of Biomedical Materials Research*, 2002. 59(3): pp. 547–556.
20. Cooke, M.N., et al., Use of stereolithography to manufacture critical-sized 3D biodegradable scaffolds for bone ingrowth. *Journal of Biomedical Materials Research Part B: Applied Biomaterials*, 2003. 64B(2): pp. 65–69.
21. Arcaute, K., B.K. Mann, and R.B. Wicker, Stereolithography of three-dimensional bioactive poly(ethylene glycol) constructs with encapsulated cells. *Annals of Biomedical Engineering*, 2006. 34(9): pp. 1429–1441.
22. Lee, K.W., et al., Poly(propylene fumarate) bone tissue engineering scaffold fabrication using stereolithography: effects of resin formulations and laser parameters. *Biomacromolecules*, 2007. 8(4): pp. 1077–1084.
23. Castro, N., P. Goldstein, and M.N. Cooke, Synthesis and manufacture of photocrosslinkable poly(caprolactone)-based three-dimensional scaffolds for tissue engineering applications. *Advances in Bioscience and Biotechnology*, 2011. 2(3): pp. 167–173.
24. Beke, S., et al., Towards excimer-laser-based stereolithography: a rapid process to fabricate rigid biodegradable photopolymer scaffolds. *Journal of the Royal Society Interface*, 2012. 9(76): pp. 3017–3026.
25. Peele, B.N., et al., 3D printing antagonistic systems of artificial muscle using projection stereolithography. *Bioinspiration & Biomimetics*, 2015. 10(5): pp. 055003.
26. Hribar, K.C., et al., Nonlinear 3D projection printing of concave hydrogel microstructures for long-term multicellular spheroid and embryoid body culture. *Lab on a Chip*, 2015. 15(11): pp. 2412–2418.
27. Grogan, S.P., et al., Digital micromirror device projection printing system for meniscus tissue engineering. *Acta Biomaterialia*, 2013. 9(7): pp. 7218–7226.
28. Lu, Y. and S. Chen, Projection printing of 3-dimensional tissue scaffolds. *Methods in Molecular Biology*, 2012. 868: pp. 289–302.
29. Melchels, F.P., J. Feijen, and D.W. Grijpma, A review on stereolithography and its applications in biomedical engineering. *Biomaterials*, 2010. 31(24): pp. 6121–6130.
30. Castro, N.J., J. O'Brien, and L.G. Zhang, Integrating biologically inspired nanomaterials and table-top stereolithography for 3D printed biomimetic osteochondral scaffolds. *Nanoscale*, 2015. 7(33): pp. 14010–14022.
31. Melchels, F.P.W., et al., Additive manufacturing of tissues and organs. *Progress in Polymer Science*, 2012. 37(8): pp. 1079–1104.
32. Cui, H., et al., Biologically inspired smart release system based on 3D bioprinted perfused scaffold for vascularized tissue regeneration. *Advanced Science*, 2016. 3(8): pp. 1–10.
33. O'Brien, C.M., et al., Three-dimensional printing of nanomaterial scaffolds for complex tissue regeneration. *Tissue Engineering: Part B*, 2015. 21(1): pp. 103–114.
34. Li, X., et al., 3D-printed biopolymers for tissue engineering application. *International Journal of Polymer Science*, 2014. 2014: pp. 1–13.
35. Holmes, B., et al., Development of novel three-dimensional printed scaffolds for osteochondral regeneration. *Tissue Engineering: Part A*, 2015. 21(1–2): pp. 403–415.
36. Liu, F.H., Y.K. Shen, and J.L. Lee, Selective laser sintering of a hydroxyapatite-silica scaffold on cultured MG63 osteoblasts in vitro. *International Journal of Precision Engineering and Manufacturing*, 2012. 13(3): pp. 439–444.
37. Long, J.P., S.J. Hollister, and S.A. Goldstein, A paradigm for the development and evaluation of novel implant topologies for bone fixation: in vivo evaluation. *Journal of Biomechanics*, 2012. 45(15): pp. 2651–2657.

38. Kang, H., et al., A paradigm for the development and evaluation of novel implant topologies for bone fixation: implant design and fabrication. *Journal of Biomechanics*, 2012. 45(13): pp. 2241–2247.

39. Rasperini, G., et al., 3D-printed bioresorbable scaffold for periodontal repair. *Journal of Dental Research*, 2015. 94(9 Suppl): pp. 153S–157S.

40. Hollister, S.J., et al., Design control for clinical translation of 3D printed modular scaffolds. *Annals of Biomedical Engineering*, 2015. 43(3): pp. 774–786.

41. Coelho, P.G., et al., Bioresorbable scaffolds for bone tissue engineering: optimal design, fabrication, mechanical testing and scale-size effects analysis. *Medical Engineering & Physics*, 2015. 37(3): pp. 287–296.

42. Liao, H.-T., J.-P. Chen, and M.-Y. Lee, Bone tissue engineering with adipose-derived stem cells in bioactive composites of laser-sintered porous polycaprolactone scaffolds and platelet-rich plasma. *Materials*, 2013. 6(11): p. 4911.

43. Liu, F.H., et al., Selective laser sintering of bio-metal scaffold. *First CIRP Conference on Biomanufacturing*, 2013. 5: pp. 83–87.

44. Lodererova, M., et al., Biocompatibility of metal sintered materials in dependence on multimaterial graded structure. *13th International Conference on Biomedical Engineering*, Vols 1–3, 2009. 23(1–3): pp. 1204–1207.

45. Hao, L., et al., Characterisation of HA/polymer bio-composite structure fabricated by selective laser sintering. *Proceedings of 3rd International Conference on Advanced Research in Virtual and Rapid Manufacturing*, Leira, Portugal, September 24–29, 2008: pp. 121–127.

46. O'Brien, C.M., et al., Three-dimensional printing of nanomaterial scaffolds for complex tissue regeneration. *Tissue Engineering Part B: Review*, 2015. 21(1): pp. 103–114.

47. Skardal, A., J. Zhang, and G.D. Prestwich, Bioprinting vessel-like constructs using hyaluronan hydrogels crosslinked with tetrahedral polyethylene glycol tetracrylates. *Biomaterials*, 2010. 31(24): pp. 6173–6181.

48. Pfister, A., et al., Biofunctional rapid prototyping for tissue-engineering applications: 3D bioplotting versus 3D printing. *Journal of Polymer Science Part A: Polymer Chemistry*, 2004. 42(3): pp. 624–638.

49. Liu, H., E.B. Slamovich, and T.J. Webster, Increased osteoblast functions among nanophase titania/poly(lactide-co-glycolide) composites of the highest nanometer surface roughness. *Journal of Biomedical Materials Research Part A*, 2006. 78(4): pp. 798–807.

50. Marszalek, J.E., et al., 2.5D constructs for characterizing phase separated polymer blend surface morphology in tissue engineering scaffolds. *Journal of Biomedical Materials Research Part A*, 2013. 101(5): pp. 1502–1510.

51. Peltola, S.M., et al., A review of rapid prototyping techniques for tissue engineering purposes. *Annals of Medicine*, 2008. 40(4): pp. 268–280.

52. Xu, T., et al., Complex heterogeneous tissue constructs containing multiple cell types prepared by inkjet printing technology. *Biomaterials*, 2013. 34(1): pp. 130–139.

53. Wust, S., R. Muller, and S. Hofmann, Controlled positioning of cells in biomaterials-approaches towards 3D tissue printing. *Journal of Functional Biomaterials*, 2011. 2(3): pp. 119–154.

54. Ferris, C.J., et al., Bio-ink for on-demand printing of living cells. *Biomaterials Science*, 2013. 1(2): pp. 224–230.

55. Buckwalter, J.A. and J.A. Martin, Osteoarthritis. *Advanced Drug Delivery Reviews*, 2006. 58(2): pp. 150–167.

56. Fontaine, K.R., S. Haaz, and M. Heo, Projected prevalence of US adults with self-reported doctor-diagnosed arthritis, 2005 to 2050. *Clinical Rheumatology*, 2007. 26(5): pp. 772–774.

57. Williams, G.M., et al., Shape, loading, and motion in the bioengineering design, fabrication, and testing of personalized synovial joints. *Journal of Biomechanics*, 2010. 43(1): pp. 156–165.

58. Thaunat, M., et al., Cartilage thickness matching of selected donor and recipient sites for osteochondral autografting of the medial femoral condyle. *Knee Surgery, Sports Traumatology, Arthroscopy,* 2007. 15(4): pp. 381–386.

59. Birman, M.V., et al., The humeral head as a potential donor source for osteochondral allograft transfer to the knee. *Journal of Knee Surgery,* 2009. 22(2): pp. 99–105.

60. Johnson, M.R. and R.F. LaPrade, Tibial plateau "Kissing Lesion" from a proud osteochondral autograft. *American Journal of Orthodontics* (Belle Mead, NJ), 2011. 40(7): pp. 359–361.

61. Temenoff, J.S. and P.J. Yang, Engineering orthopedic tissue interfaces. *Tissue Engineering Part B: Reviews,* 2009. 15(2): pp. 127–141.

62. Hutmacher, D.W., Scaffolds in tissue engineering bone and cartilage. *Biomaterials,* 2000. 21(24): pp. 2529–2543.

63. Zhang, L., J. Hu, and K.A. Athanasiou, The role of tissue engineering in articular cartilage repair and regeneration. *Critical Reviews in Biomedical Engineering,* 2009. 37(1–2): pp. 1–57.

64. Chen, J., et al., Simultaneous regeneration of articular cartilage and subchondral bone in vivo using MSCs induced by a spatially controlled gene delivery system in bilayered integrated scaffolds. *Biomaterials,* 2011. 32(21): pp. 4793–4805.

65. Guo, X., et al., Repair of osteochondral defects with biodegradable hydrogel composites encapsulating marrow mesenchymal stem cells in a rabbit model. *Acta Biomaterialia,* 2010. 6(1): pp. 39–47.

66. Fedorovich, N.E., et al., Biofabrication of osteochondral tissue equivalents by printing topologically defined, cell-laden hydrogel scaffolds. *Tissue Engineering Part C: Methods,* 2012. 18(1): pp. 33–44.

67. Gao, G., et al., Inkjet-bioprinted acrylated peptides and PEG hydrogel with human mesenchymal stem cells promote robust bone and cartilage formation with minimal printhead clogging. *Biotechnology Journal,* 2015. 10(10): pp. 1568–1577.

68. Castro, N.J., C.M. O'Brien, and L.G. Zhang, Biomimetic biphasic 3-D nanocomposite scaffold for osteochondral regeneration. *AIChE Journal,* 2014. 60(2): pp. 432–442.

69. Castro, N.J., J. O'Brien, and L.G. Zhang, Integrating biologically inspired nanomaterials and table-top stereolithography for 3D printed biomimetic osteochondral scaffolds. *Nanoscale,* 2015. 7(33): pp. 14010–14022.

70. Zhang, W., et al., Cartilage repair and subchondral bone migration using 3D printing osteochondral composites: a one-year-period study in rabbit trochlea. *BioMed Research International,* 2014. 2014: p. 746138.

71. Shim, J.H., et al., Three-dimensional bioprinting of multilayered constructs containing human mesenchymal stromal cells for osteochondral tissue regeneration in the rabbit knee joint. *Biofabrication,* 2016. 8(1): p. 014102.

72. Jain, R.K. and P. Carmeliet, Angiogenesis in cancer and other diseases. *Nature,* 2000. 407(6801): pp. 249–257.

73. Rouwkema, J., N.C. Rivron, and C.A. van Blitterswijk, Vascularization in tissue engineering. *Trends in Biotechnology,* 2008. 26(8): pp. 434–441.

74. Druecke, D., et al., Neovascularization of poly(ether ester) block-copolymer scaffolds in vivo: long-term investigations using intravital fluorescent microscopy. *Journal of Biomedical Materials Research Part A,* 2004. 68A(1): pp. 10–18.

75a. Kolesky, D.B., et al., Three-dimensional bioprinting of thick vascularized tissues. *Proceedings of the National Academy of Sciences,* 2016. 113(12): pp. 3179–3184.

75b. Kolesky, D.B., et al., 3D bioprinting of vascularized, heterogeneous cell-laden tissue constructs. *Advanced Materials,* 2014. 26(19): pp. 3124–3130.

76. Paulsen, S.J. and J.S. Miller, Tissue vascularization through 3D printing: will technology bring us flow? *Developmental Dynamics,* 2015. 244(5): pp. 629–640.

77. Cui, H., et al., Hierarchical fabrication of engineered vascularized bone biphasic constructs via dual 3D bioprinting: integrating regional bioactive factors into architectural design. *Advanced Healthcare Materials*, 2016. 5(17): pp. 2174–2181.

78. Irons, H.R., et al., Three-dimensional neural constructs: a novel platform for neurophysiological investigation. *Journal of Neural Engineering*, 2008. 5(3): pp. 333–341.

79. Ma, W., et al., CNS stem and progenitor cell differentiation into functional neuronal circuits in three-dimensional collagen gels. *Experimental Neurology*, 2004. 190(2): pp. 276–288.

80. Li, N., et al., Three-dimensional graphene foam as a biocompatible and conductive scaffold for neural stem cells. *Scientific Reports*, 2013. 3: p. 1604.

81. Lee, Y.B., et al., Bio-printing of collagen and VEGF-releasing fibrin gel scaffolds for neural stem cell culture. *Experimental Neurology*, 2010. 223(2): pp. 645–652.

82. Lozano, R., et al., 3D printing of layered brain-like structures using peptide modified gellan gum substrates. *Biomaterials*, 2015. 67: pp. 264–273.

83. Xu, T., et al., Viability and electrophysiology of neural cell structures generated by the inkjet printing method. *Biomaterials*, 2006. 27(19): pp. 3580–3588.

84. Hsieh, F.Y., H.H. Lin, and S.H. Hsu, 3D bioprinting of neural stem cell-laden thermoresponsive biodegradable polyurethane hydrogel and potential in central nervous system repair. *Biomaterials*, 2015. 71: pp. 48–57.

85. Lee, S.-J., et al., Development of novel 3D printed scaffolds with core-shell nanoparticles for nerve regeneration. *IEEE Transactions on Biomedical Engineering*, 2017. 64(2): pp. 1–1.

86. Weng, B., et al., Inkjet printed polypyrrole/collagen scaffold: a combination of spatial control and electrical stimulation of PC12 cells. *Synthetic Metals*, 2012. 162(15–16): pp. 1375–1380.

87. Jakus, A.E., et al., Three-dimensional printing of high-content graphene scaffolds for electronic and biomedical applications. *ACS Nano*, 2015. 9(4): pp. 4636–4648.

88. Tse, C., et al., Inkjet printing Schwann cells and neuronal analogue NG108-15 cells. *Biofabrication*, 2016. 8(1): p. 015017.

89. Gao, B., et al., 4D bioprinting for biomedical applications. *Trends in Biotechnology*, 2016. 34(9): pp. 746–756.

90. Galaev, I.Y. and B. Mattiasson, "Smart" polymers and what they could do in biotechnology and medicine. *Trends in Biotechnology*, 1999. 17(8): pp. 335–340.

91. Kokkinis, D., M. Schaffner, and A.R. Studart, Multimaterial magnetically assisted 3D printing of composite materials. *Nature Communications*, 2015. 6: p. 8643.

92. Sydney Gladman, A., et al., Biomimetic 4D printing. *Nature Materials*, 2016. 15(4): p. 413.

93. Miao, S., et al., 4D printing smart biomedical scaffolds with novel soybean oil epoxidized acrylate. *Scientific Reports*, 2016. 6: p. 27226.

94. Neuss, S., et al., The use of a shape-memory poly(ε-caprolactone)dimethacrylate network as a tissue engineering scaffold. *Biomaterials*, 2009. 30(9): pp. 1697–1705.

95. Lendlein, A. and S. Kelch, Shape-memory polymers. *Angewandte Chemie-International Edition*, 2002. 41(12): pp. 2034–2057.

CHAPTER 8

Regenerative Engineering of the Human Using Convergence

Cato T. Laurencin

University of Connecticut Health Center; Raymond and Beverly Sackler Center for Biomedical, Biological, Physical and Engineering Sciences; University of Connecticut

Naveen Nagiah

University of Connecticut Health Center

CONTENTS

Musculoskeletal injuries are common in America. It is now estimated that over 99 million ambulatory visits for musculoskeletal injuries take place each year in the United States, and by all accounts that number is continuing to grow. At this point, 77% of injuries that require a doctor's visit are musculoskeletal (1). The price of musculoskeletal injuries is very high. Over 100 billion dollars in direct costs are spent each year (1). These numbers do not consider indirect costs such as lost wages from disability or recuperation post surgery. Thus, these injuries represent a significant health concern in America and, indeed, throughout the world.

The field of tissue engineering can be described as the application of biological, chemical, and engineering principles toward the repair, restoration, or regeneration of living tissues using materials, cells, and factors alone or in combination (2). Dr. Laurencin first presented this definition almost 20 years ago and it has stood the test of time. The field began approximately 30 years ago, when Dr. Y. C. Fung first coined the term "tissue engineering."

The field has undergone some changes but has substantially kept to the original themes surrounding it. But while the field of tissue engineering has been largely unchanged, science and technology have changed along with our understanding of the importance of bringing together technologies to be able to truly make leapfrog-type advances in the engineering of tissues. Several substantive changes that include new technologies that were absent in tissue engineering research were born and are rapidly expanding far beyond the encompassed fields in tissue engineering.

8.1 HISTORY OF REGENERATIVE ENGINEERING

In the early 2000s, Dr. Laurencin began to discuss the fact that perhaps we should be thinking about a new way to approach the engineering of tissues, one that would embrace newer technologies and create a bigger tent for the process of regeneration. At meetings such as the Keystone Meeting and the Society for Biomaterials Grand Challenges meetings, he suggested that this new way of thinking about engineering tissues could be called "Regenerative Engineering."

As the vision was developed, the editors of *Science Magazine* discussed with Dr. Laurencin the approach to thinking about the future of Tissue Engineering. In a landmark piece in *Science Translational Medicine*, Dr. Laurencin provided his vision of the future of tissue engineering in a publication produced with Professor Yusuf Khan titled "Regenerative Engineering." The piece spoke to the fact that the future of engineering lies in a new field called regenerative engineering and that biomaterial science and engineering would play an important role in the development of this field.

The definition of regenerative engineering has undergone slight modifications over time but has stayed true to the notion that it is a Convergence field (3). By this, we mean that it is a field that brings together many new fields and works together to create new ways of thinking and new technologies. Regenerative Engineering capitalizes on relying on science and technology areas that are new areas that we did not possess during the period of time in which tissue engineering was first born. We define regenerative engineering as the convergence of the advanced materials science, stem cell science, physics, developmental biology, and clinical translation toward the regeneration of complex tissues, organs, and organ systems. As we have discussed, Regenerative Engineering can be viewed as a true Convergence field where the coming together of insights and approaches from originally distinct fields fuels the work done in Regenerative Engineering (Figure 8.1).

The concept of convergence as bringing together areas of biology, biomedicine, engineering, and physics was described by Professors Phil Sharp and Robert Langer in their important publication on the subject just a few years ago (3). It is these areas of advanced materials science, stem cell science, physics, developmental biology, and clinical translation that really define this new area that we call regenerative engineering. The emphasis is on newer tools and technologies that appear disparate and are not utilized in traditional schools of thought in engineering tissues (such as physics and developmental biology). This chapter discusses aspects of the use of regenerative engineering technologies, techniques, and approaches for the regeneration of bone and soft tissue.

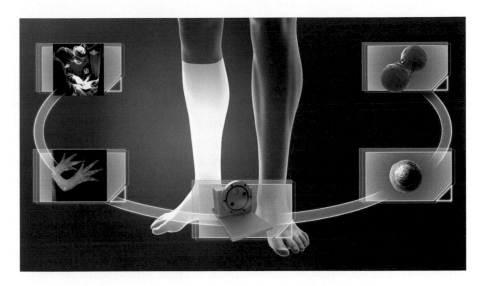

FIGURE 8.1   Convergence of various fields for whole limb regeneration.

8.2 REGENERATIVE ENGINEERING FOR BONE DEFECTS

Ideal bone scaffolds should be designed to fit the area of defect and heal only the area of the defect without affecting the surrounding healthy tissue. Sintered biocompatible, uniform, smooth polymer microspheres were chosen initially to fill these defects, as illustrated in Figure 8.2. Polymer microspheres of uniform size distribution with smooth surfaces can be controlling parameters via polymer concentration, stirring speed, and surfactant concentration.

Sintering of the polymer microsphere matrices to a desired dimension and shape can be achieved by packing of the microspheres in the desired volume of the mold and heating them to a temperature slightly above the glass transition temperature of the polymer(s). The growth of healthy tissue on the polymer surface and between them will ensure complete healing at the defect site. The rate of degradation of the polymer microspheres can be modulated with respect to the rate of healing to enable complete closure at the defect site at the end of the healing process. The mechanical properties of the sintered microsphere

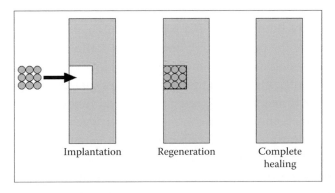

FIGURE 8.2   Sintered polymer microspheres for complete healing of bone defects.

matrix should also be relatable to the native bone properties for enhanced regeneration in the defect site. Based on the diameter of the microspheres, the compressive modulus of the scaffold can be altered. The microsphere diameter inversely varies with the compressive properties of the sintered scaffold. Based on their diameter, mechanical properties ranging from 250-MPa compressive modulus to approximately 500-MPa compressive modulus were developed. These matrices were implanted in *in vivo* rabbit models with surgically created ulnar defects. The rabbit model is an excellent model to study bone regeneration as the radius bone on the opposite side acts as an internal strut allowing for partial load bearing of the sintered microspheres polymer matrix inside the bone defect. The effect of sintered polymer microspheres loaded with the growth factor bone morphogenetic protein (BMP) in conjunction with bone marrow-derived stem cells on bone regeneration was studied. Bone marrow-derived stem cells are fibroblastic-like in shape and can differentiate along multiple lineages, such as osteoblasts, chondrocytes, adipocytes, and hematopoiesis-supportive stroma (4). This combination demonstrated its effectiveness when the critical bone defect was filled with regenerated healthy tissue, which otherwise would not occur naturally as observed on the other ulna without sintered microspheres implants. The presence of BMP and bone marrow-derived stem cells were found to enhance the healing. Bone formation along the surface of the sintered polymeric microspheres and vasculature along the matrix was also observed. Hence, sintered polymer microspheres with tunable mechanical properties and size, when used in conjunction with BMP and bone marrow stromal cells, proved to be a translational scaffold for enhanced regeneration of defects in bone tissue. The success of the polymer microspheres has inspired the production of a myriad polymer microspheres and its blends encapsulated with different cytokines for enhanced and healthy regeneration of defective bone. To bridge developmental biology and stem cell science with engineering approaches, a multitude of stem cell sources have been isolated and its effectiveness in bone formation has been analyzed. After considerable research, adipose-derived stem cells are considered to be an important source for regeneration capability due to their ease of isolation, processability, and abundance of accessibility from the donor (5). Moreover, its multipotency to differentiate into a desired cell type, including cartilage and bone depending on the presence of growth factors, has been exploited. Polymer microspheres coated or encapsulated with ceramic systems have also been developed. The combination of polymer microspheres and ceramics can potentially be the ideal interface by providing the best of both worlds. The polymer matrix is versatile in the creation of porous structures while the ceramic component of the scaffolds can provide the stiffness of the scaffold, thereby enhancing the mechanical stability of the scaffold. Based on the composition of the ceramic material in the combination system, the mechanical properties of the material can be tuned for site-specific mechanical functionality and regeneration. Moreover, the ceramics being inorganic in nature can trigger osteoinductive pathways if properly formulated, meaning the stem cells can be differentiated to the osteogenic phenotype based on the mechanical and physical cues provided by the ceramics. A series of studies based on polymer-ceramic composite microspheres have demonstrated different release patterns of calcium ions from their respective systems. Polymer matrices alone have shown no release of calcium ions from its matrix while increasing the low crystalline ceramic

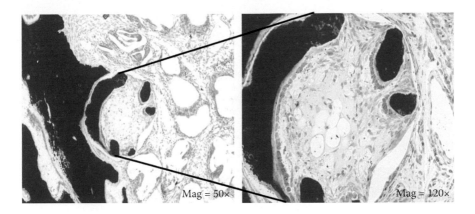

FIGURE 8.3   H & E staining of critical size bone defect healing with osteoinductive matrices (6).

concentration in the composition of the scaffold system has shown a concurrent release of calcium ions from its composite system. The ceramic composition was found to play a pivotal role in increasing the release of calcium in the composite system. *In vivo* studies conducted with rats and rabbits with critical size bone defects have amply demonstrated the osteoinductive ability of these composite scaffolds to subsequent bone regeneration. Figure 8.3 represents a histology section after 8 weeks of implantation. Evidence of remodeling and healing is clearly observed after 8 weeks of implantation in the callus of the composite scaffold. Multinucleated osteoclasts are seen along the border between the fibrous tissue and the mineralized tissue. The physiochemical cues provided by these composite matrices have greatly reduced the use of expensive cytokines and growth factors like BMP. In addition, ceramic-polymer composite matrices have the potential of drastically reducing the cost of scaffold production and maintenance until use.

With the onset of nanotechnology, nanospheres were synthesized and were observed to have the potential of also demonstrating regenerative capability when polymers and ceramics are combined. Current studies are under way to investigate the immense potential of these polymer nanospheres with ceramics for enhanced regeneration of the defects in bone.

8.3 REGENERATIVE ENGINEERING FOR ANTERIOR CRUCIATE LIGAMENT REGENERATION

We have examined the use of regenerative engineering technologies for the regeneration of the anterior cruciate ligament (ACL). The ACL is the major intraarticular ligament of the knee, which is responsible for angular motion stability and acts as an overall stabilizer of the knee. Injuries or tears to the ligament lead to excessive joint mobility and instability of the knee. Due to its intricate structure and functionality, regeneration of a completely healed and functioning ligament after injury is a major challenge mandating the need for surgical intervention. Figure 8.4 shows the fibrous hierarchical design of the ACL (7). The ACL consists predominantly of fiber bundles. Collagen fibrils form fiber bundles which are further grouped into fascicles with a specific orientation. The arrangement of the fascicles within the ligament vary from being thick and dense to small and loosely

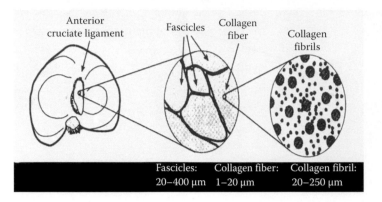

FIGURE 8.4   ACL fibrous hierarchical design (7).

embedded. Similarly, the orientation of the fascicles is helical in the sides and parallel in the center. This results in varying load bearing capacity of the fascicles according to the varying knee motion (7). The scaffold designed for ACL regeneration must mimic the fibrous structure of the ACL at the microstructural level with a comparable load bearing capacity to the native ACL.

Polymer filaments with textile structure can mimic the microstructural morphology of the ACL collagen fibrils. The textile structures can be braided or interwoven together to obtain highly porous structures for tissue infiltration with enhanced impact resistance. The structure also aids in transferring high loads with an innate ability for structural elongation. Figure 8.5 shows a braided polymer filament to fibrous scaffolds with different interphases mimicking the fascicles structure in the ACL designed by Dr. Laurencin and his team. The ability to create new structural braids allows for the tailoring of mechanical

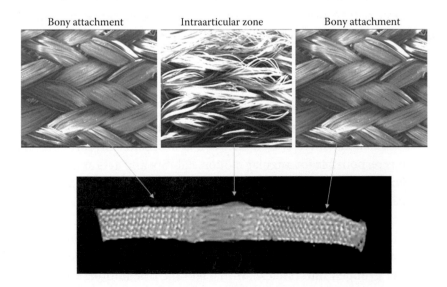

FIGURE 8.5   Custom-designed braided polymer filaments mimicking ACL microstructure (8).

properties required for regeneration. The two ends of the textile scaffolds were fabricated to mimic the bony attachments on either side of the ligament while an intermediate section consists of fibers meant to mimic the connective soft tissue with no braids. *In vitro* studies showed infiltration and complete attachment of cells on the surface of the scaffolds and suggested a high translational ability of the textile structured scaffolds. *In vivo* studies in rabbit models resulted in new ACL ligamentous tissue rich in collagen type I after 3 months of surgical reconstruction.

8.4 REGENERATIVE ENGINEERING FOR ROTATOR CUFF INJURY

Another area of importance in the musculoskeletal arena involves exploring the role of regenerative engineering for rotator cuff injury treatments. Shoulder pain is a common symptom characterized by persistent and often disabling pain in the upper extremity and affects nearly 18%–26% of adults (9). Rotator cuff tears contribute to the debilitating joint injuries and are more pronounced in aging populations (9). The failure of improper healing and regeneration of original tissue characterized by tendon retraction and fatty expansion of rotator cuff muscle is the root cause for surgical failures in treating rotator cuff tears (10). Recurrent and chronic irreparable rotator cuff tears can lead to limited pain management and therapeutic ineffectiveness by all of the above-mentioned methods necessitating surgical intervention. An ideal matrix for treatment must exhibit an optimized stiffness modulus and ultimate load combined with optimal suture retention properties (11). Similar to the microspheres-based systems, polymer systems, polymer-growth factor systems, polymer-cell systems, and combination systems with convergence have been used (12–15). One other system unique to the regeneration of the rotator cuff includes a polymer-physical system wherein a cyclic strain in a custom-designed bioreactor was used to enhance the growth of cells on the polymer *in vitro* (16). In recent years, electrospun fibrous mats mimicking the native extracellular matrix have been studied for various tissue regeneration applications. The ease of processing, in addition to its versatility of spinning myriad polymer and composite fibrous structures from a few nanometers to microns, has enabled the production of a large array of materials being produced through the electrospinning process. Figure 8.6 presents the scaffold loaded with mesenchymal stem cells for rotator cuff regeneration. *In vivo* studies of mesenchymal stem cells-loaded electrospun fibers have demonstrated immense potential for translation in humans (16).

Current trends in regenerative engineering research are significantly increasing the possibility that engineered matrices which provide for mechanical augmentation over the course of healing can be clinically employed. Although smart biomaterials of natural, synthetic, blended, and composite origin have been widely examined, most studies are still restricted to smaller animal models. A convergence of deeper and better understanding of developmental biology, biological chemistry, and molecular level interactions that govern cellular behavior to direct stem cells to emulate the process of tissue development, differentiation, and growth of complete and complex multicellular tissues is really the goal.

This new field "Regenerative Engineering" is the convergence of advanced materials science, stem cell science, physics, developmental biology, and clinical translation to answer the grand challenge, i.e., to regenerate complex multicellular organs. The optimal matrix

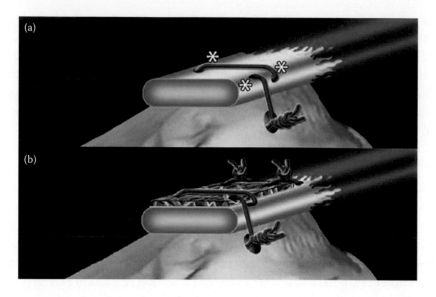

FIGURE 8.6 Non-augmented and augmented rat supraspinatus repair model. (a) Modified Mason Allen stitch. Purple indicates suture, ∗ indicates areas of stress. (b) Integrated matrix augmentation model for supraspinatus tendon repair. Green indicates the side of cell seeding in the polymer-cell group (16).

design may combine different biomaterials, consisting of mineral gradients mimicking extracellular structures with controlled biological factors eluting materials with resemblance to the natural tissue. We are now at the precipice of understanding how physical forces can influence the cellular responses taking place through our developing expertise in mechanobiology. Unlocking cues from developmental biology will hold an important key to bringing leapfrog approaches to regenerating complex tissues.

REFERENCES

1. Cullen, K.A., Hall, M.J., and Golosinskiy, A. 2009. Ambulatory surgery in the United States, 2006. National Health Statistics Report Number 11, 1–28.
2. Laurencin, C.T. and Khan, Y. 2012. Regenerative engineering. *Sci. Transl. Med.* 4, 160ed9.
3. Sharp, P.A. and Langer, R. 2011. Promoting convergence in biomedical science. *Science* 333, 527.
4. Derubeis, A.R. and Cancedda, R. 2004. Bone marrow stromal cells (BMSCs) in bone engineering: Limitations and recent advances. *Ann. Biomed. Eng.* 32, 160–165.
5. Bunnell, B.A., Flaat, M., Gagliardi, C., Patel, B., and Ripoll, C. 2008. Adipose-derived stem cells: Isolation, expansion and differentiation. *Methods* 45, 115–120.
6. Cushnie, E.K., Ulery, B.D., Nelson, S.J., Deng, M., Sethuraman, S., Doty, S.B., Lo, K.W.H., Khan, Y.M., and Laurencin, C.T. 2014. Simple signaling molecules for inductive bone regenerative engineering. *PLoS One* 9(7), e101627.
7. Jackson, D.W., Heinrich, J.T., and Simon, T. 1994. Biologic and synthetic implants to replace the anterior cruciate ligament. *Arthroscopy* 10, 442–452.
8. Cooper, J.A., Lu, H.H., Ko, F., Freeman, J.W., and Laurencin, C.T. 2005. Fiber-based tissue-engineered scaffold for ligament replacement: Design considerations and in vitro evaluation. *Biomaterials* 26, 1523–1532.
9. Linaker, C.H. and Bone W.K. 2015. Shoulder disorders and occupation. *Best Pract. Res. Clin. Rheumatol.* 29, 405–423.

10. Ricchetti, E.T., Aurora, A., Iannotti, J.P., and Derwin, K.A. 2012. Scaffold devices for rotator cuff repair. *J Shoulder Elbow Surg.* 21, 251–265.
11. Lipner, J., Cavinatto, L., Liu, W., Havlioglu, N., Xia. Y., Galatz, L.M., and Thomopoulos, S. 2015. In vivo evaluation of adipose-derived stromal cells delivered with a nanofiber scaffold for tendon-to-bone repair. *Tissue Eng. Part A* 21, 2766–2774.
12. Snyder, S., Bond, J., and Dopirak, R. 2007. Arthroscopic total rotator cuff replacement with an acellular human dermal allograft matrix. *Int. J. Shoulder Surg.* 1, 7–15.
13. Yang, G., Lin, H., Rothrauff, B.B, Yu, S., and Tuan, R.S. 2016. Multilayered polycaprolactone/gelatin fiber-hydrogel composite for tendon tissue engineering. *Acta Biomater.* 35, 68–76.
14. Tokunaga, T., Ide, J., and Arimura, H. 2015. Local application of gelatin hydrogel sheets impregnated with platelet-derived growth factor bb promotes tendon-to-bone healing after rotator cuff repair in rats. *Arthroscopy* 31, 1482–1491.
15. Grier, W.K., Moy, A.S., and Harley, B.A.C. 2017. Cyclic tensile strain enhances human mesenchymal stem cell Smad 2/3 activation and tenogenic differentiation in anisotropic collagen-glycosaminoglycan scaffolds. *Euro. Cells Mat.* 33, 227–239.
16. Peach, M.S., Ramos, D.M., James, R., Morozowich, N.L, Mazzocca, A.D., Doty, S.B, Kumbar, S., and Laurencin, C.T. 2017. Engineered stem cell niche matrices for rotator cuff tendon regenerative engineering. *PLoS One* 12, 4, e0174789.

Index